Mandalas for Mindfulness
Volume 2

31 Mandalas & Inspirational Quotes

Adult Coloring Book for Relief from Stress, Anxiety & Depression

By Nerine Martin
ColorYourWayToHappy.com

Cover and Book Design by Nerine Martin

www.ColorYourWayToHappy.com

Preview of Designs Inside This Book

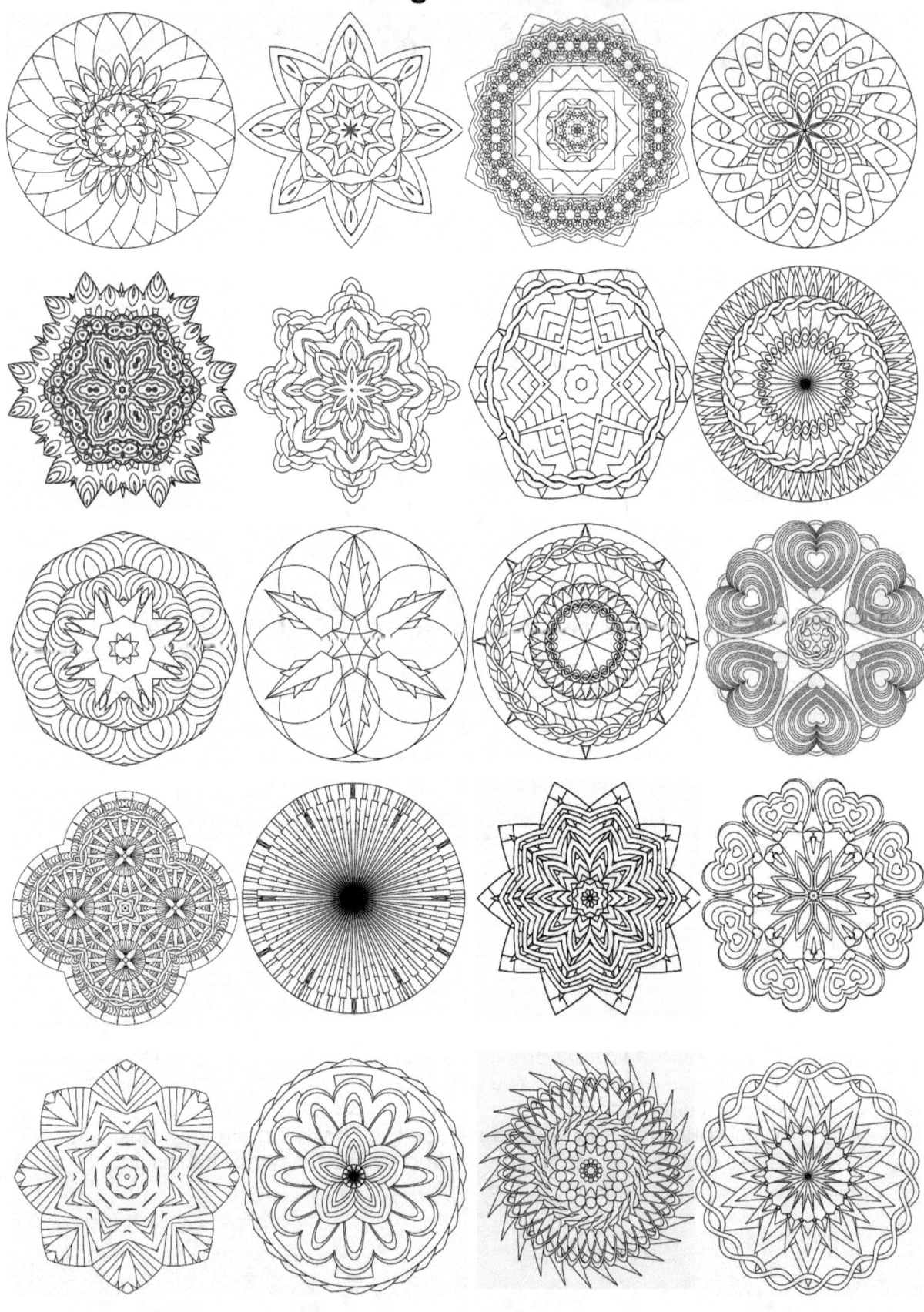

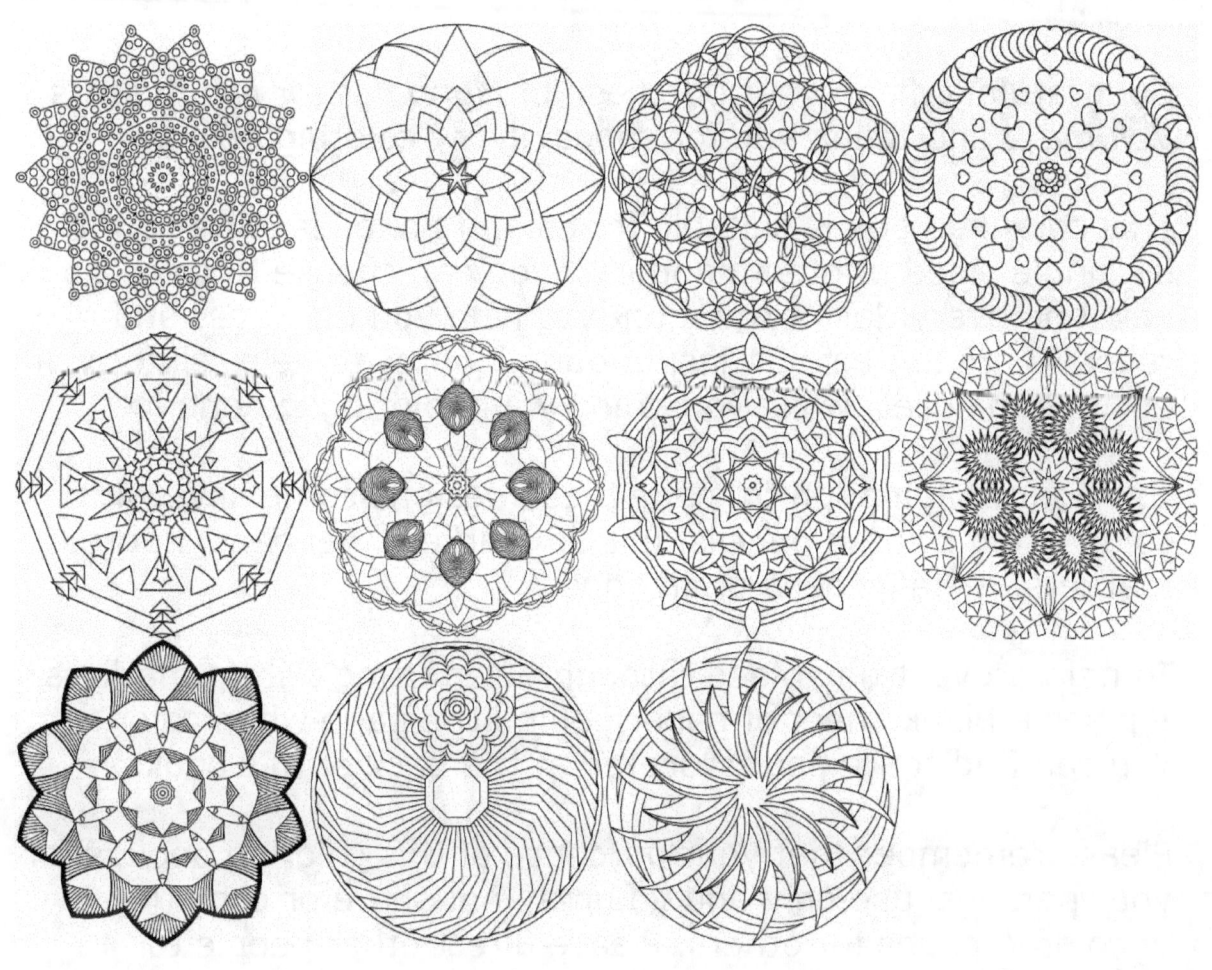

Congratulations on your purchase of *Mandalas for Mindfulness Volume 2* and thank you for choosing my coloring book.

This coloring book is suitable for colorers of all levels and with 31 single sided printed mandalas, you can choose to color a new one every day of the month to help you de-stress and relax. There are also 31 inspirational quotes to help reinforce a positive mindset, while you enjoy your coloring experience.

Use your imagination to make these designs come alive with color, using colored pencils, felt tip markers, gel pens, fluoro markers, metallic pens or crayons.

To help prevent any bleed through when using felt tip markers – place a blank sheet of paper behind the page when coloring. You can find spare pages located at the back of this book.

Please remember that your purchase of this coloring book is for your personal use only and you may not share or copy the uncolored pages for others. Please direct other people to purchase their own copy. By doing so, you are supporting my art so I can continue to make more coloring books and I thank you for your understanding and support. ☺

I hope you enjoy coloring my book and that you 'Color Your Way To Happy'.

Yours in coloring,

Nerine ☺

P.S. If you enjoy this coloring book, please be so kind to leave a review on Amazon.

Use This Area To Test Your Colors

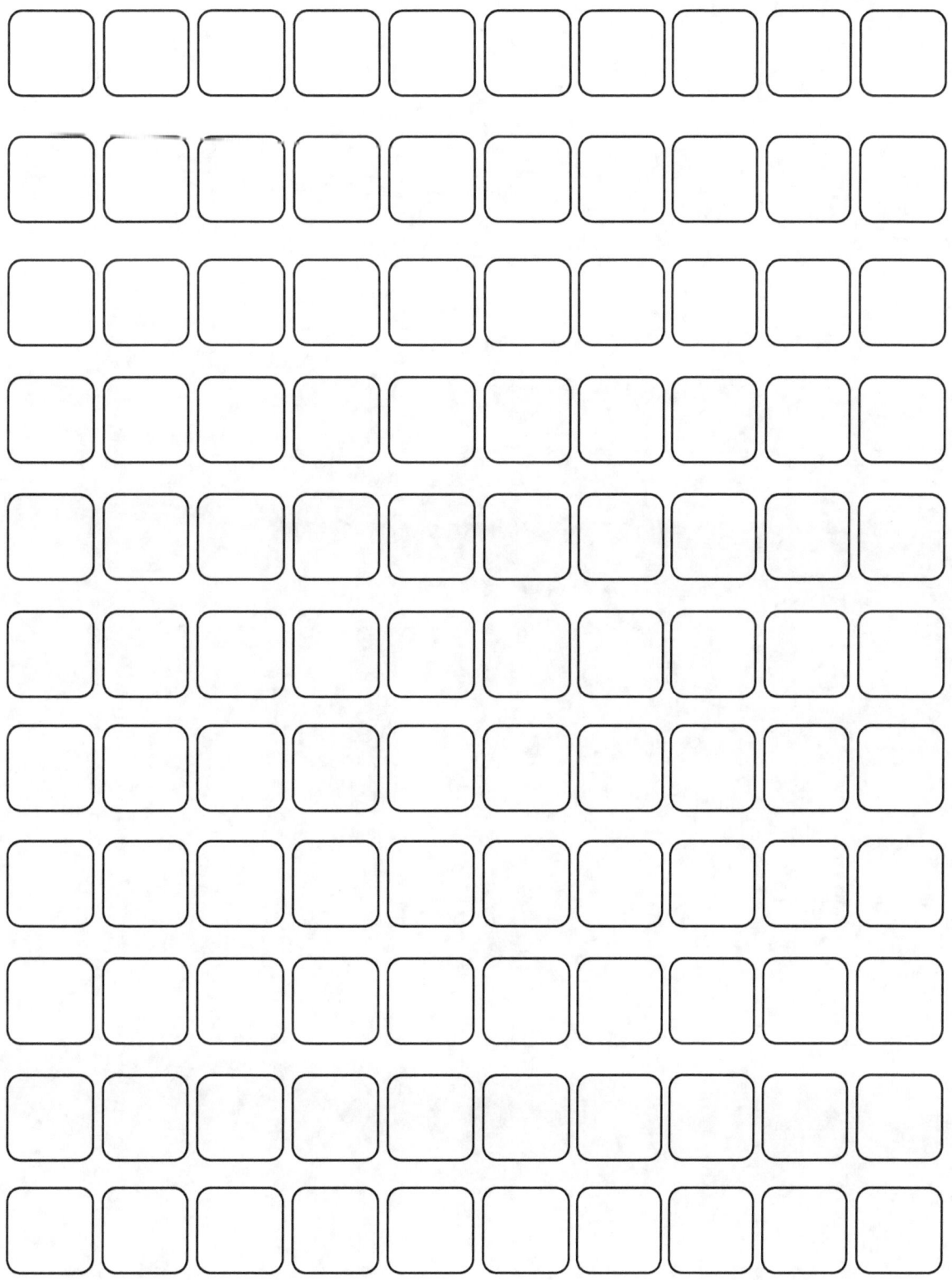

Use This Area To Try Your Colors

Live every moment
Laugh every day
Love beyond words

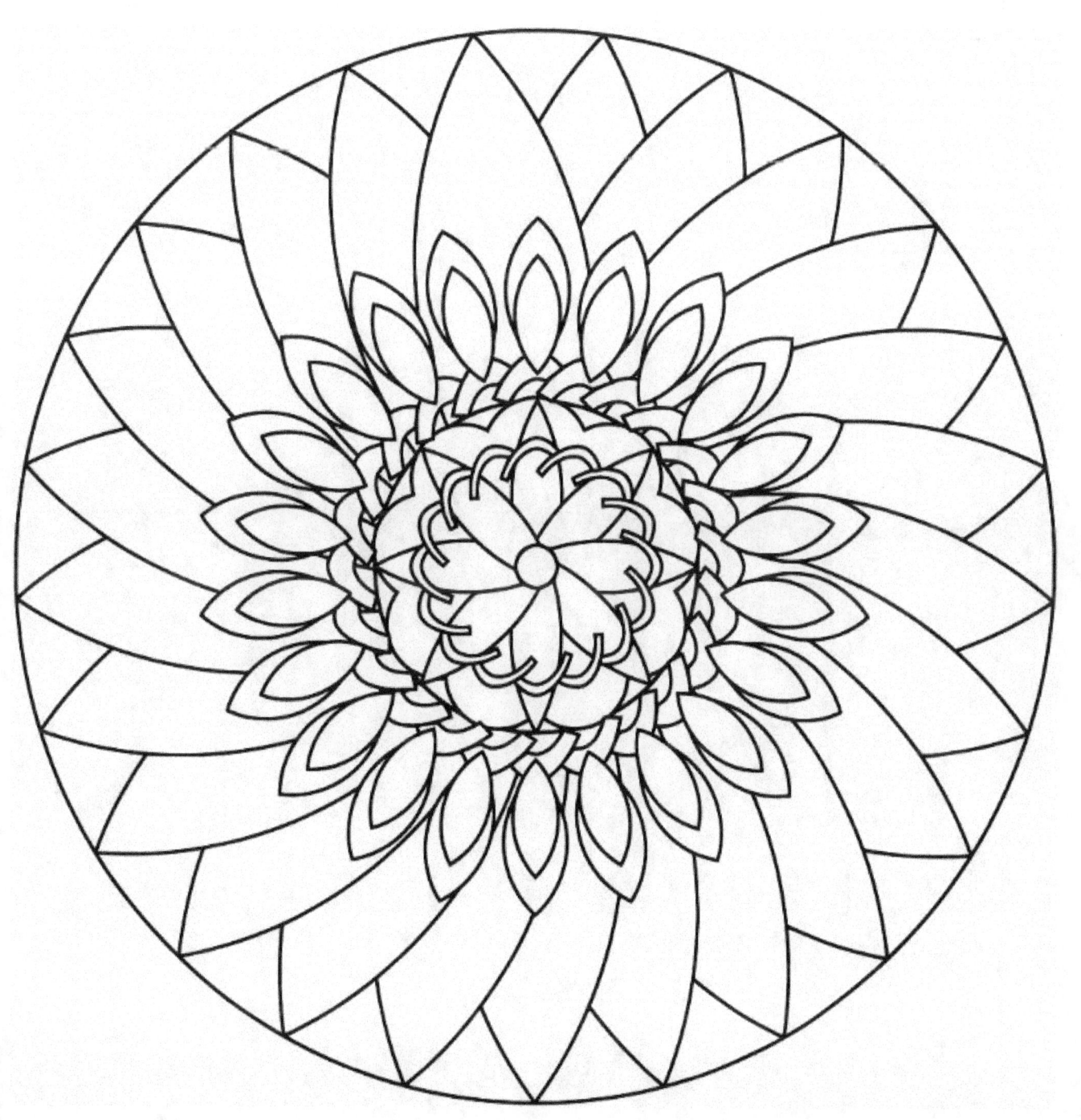

"Happiness depends upon ourselves."

Aristotle

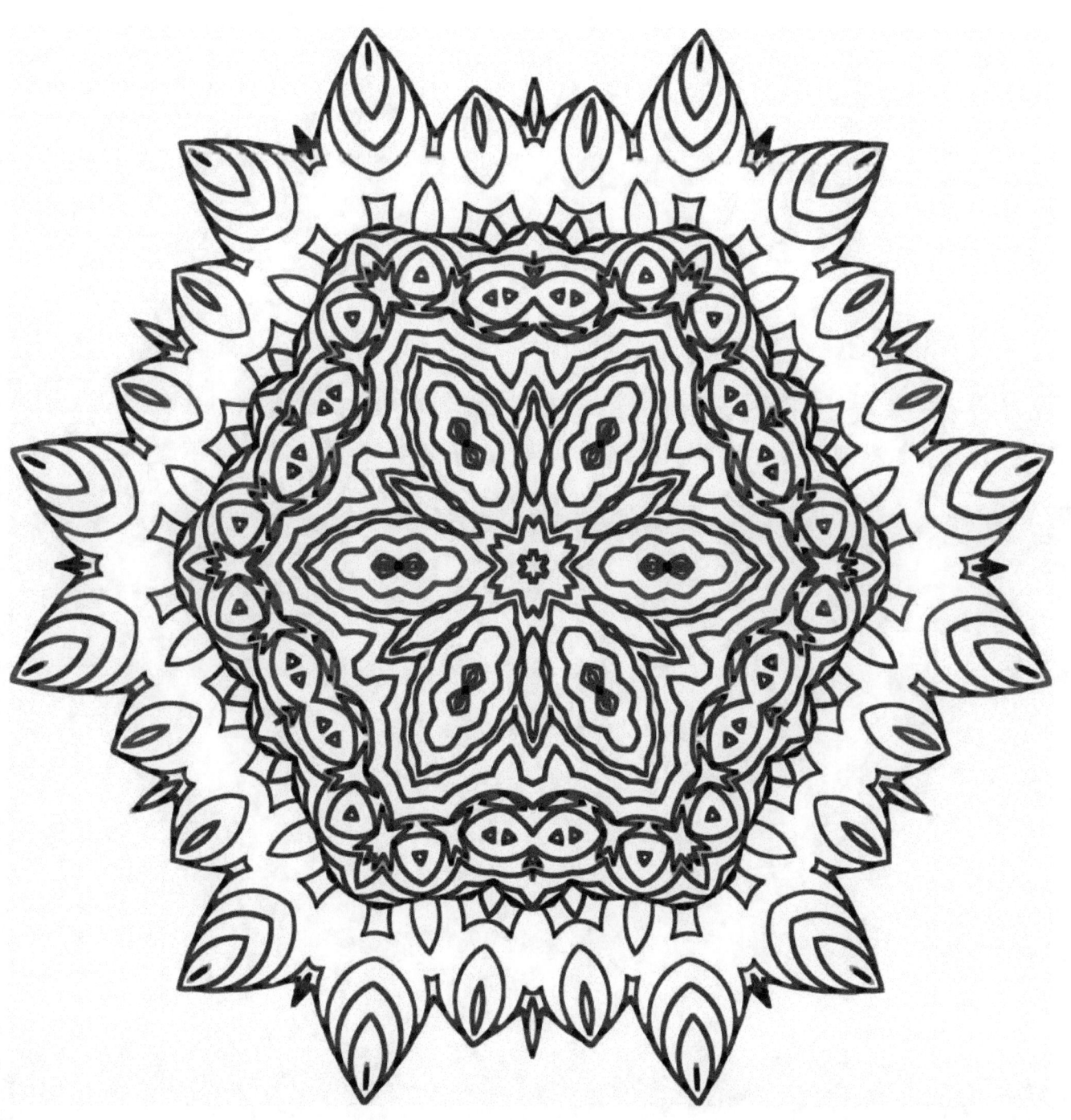

"A man is but the product
of his thoughts.
What he thinks, he
becomes."

Mohandas Karamchand
Gandhi

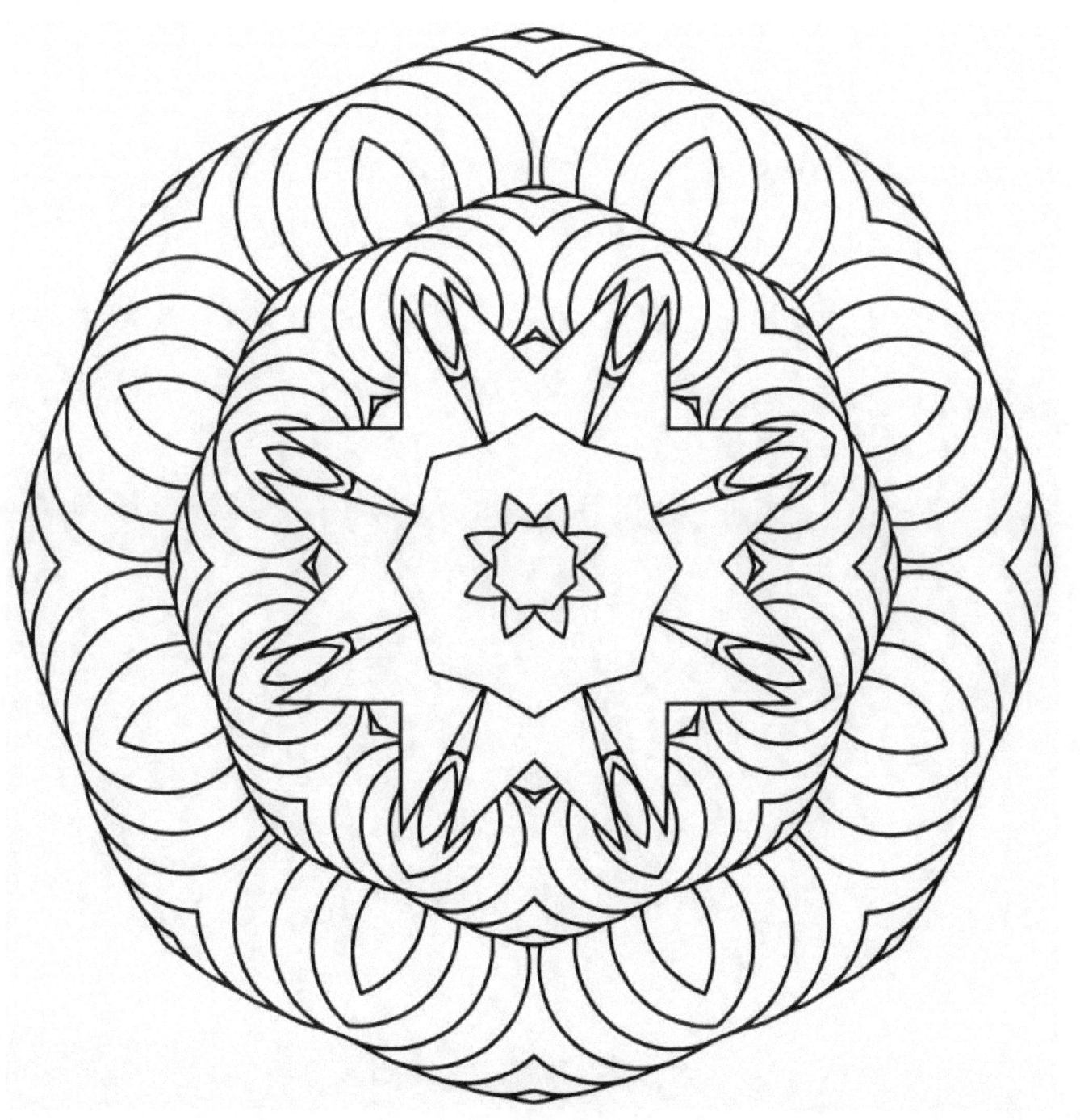

You will only be as happy,
as you make up your
mind to be!

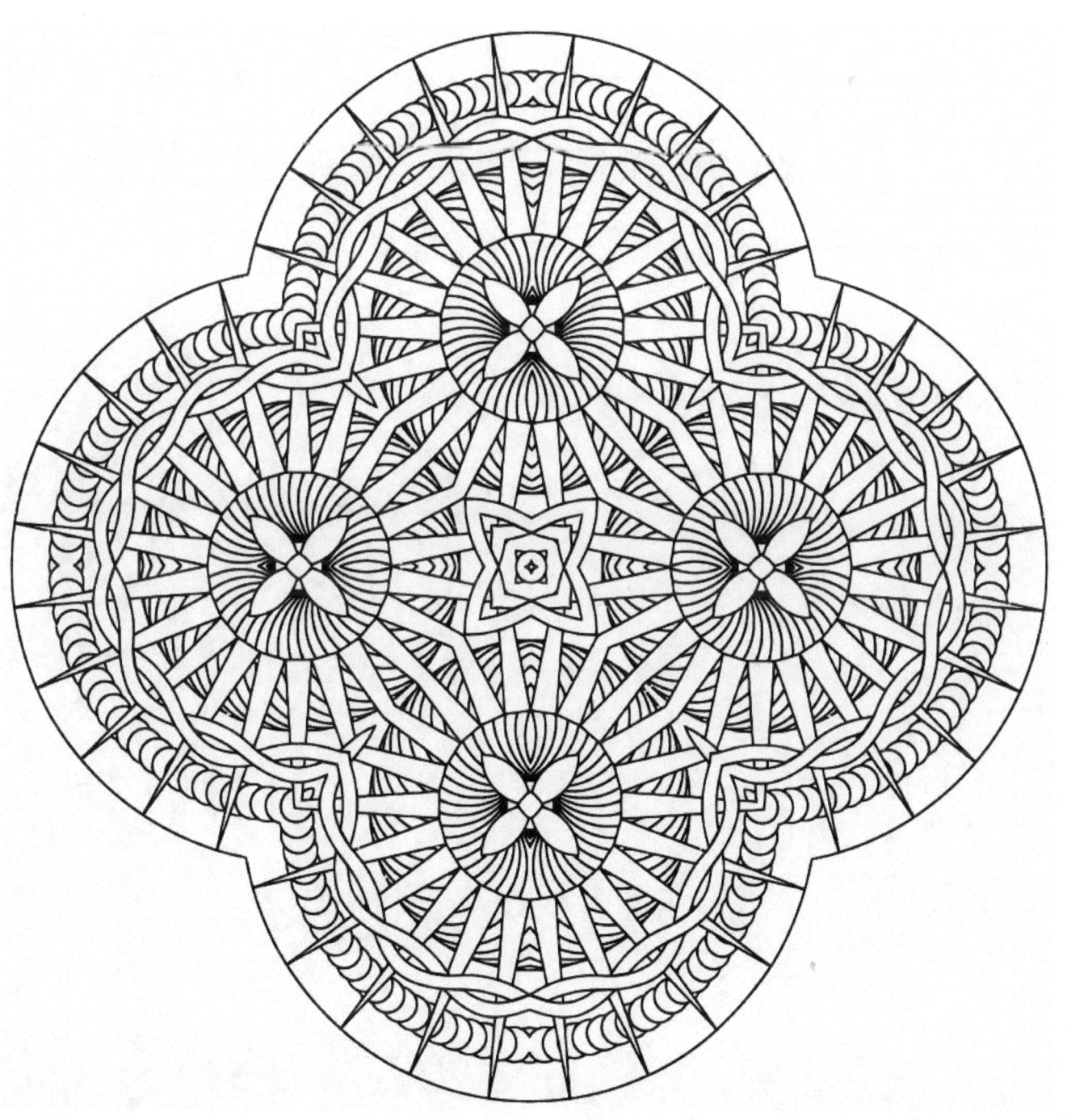

*Practice thinking good
thoughts and
you will attract more of
them!*

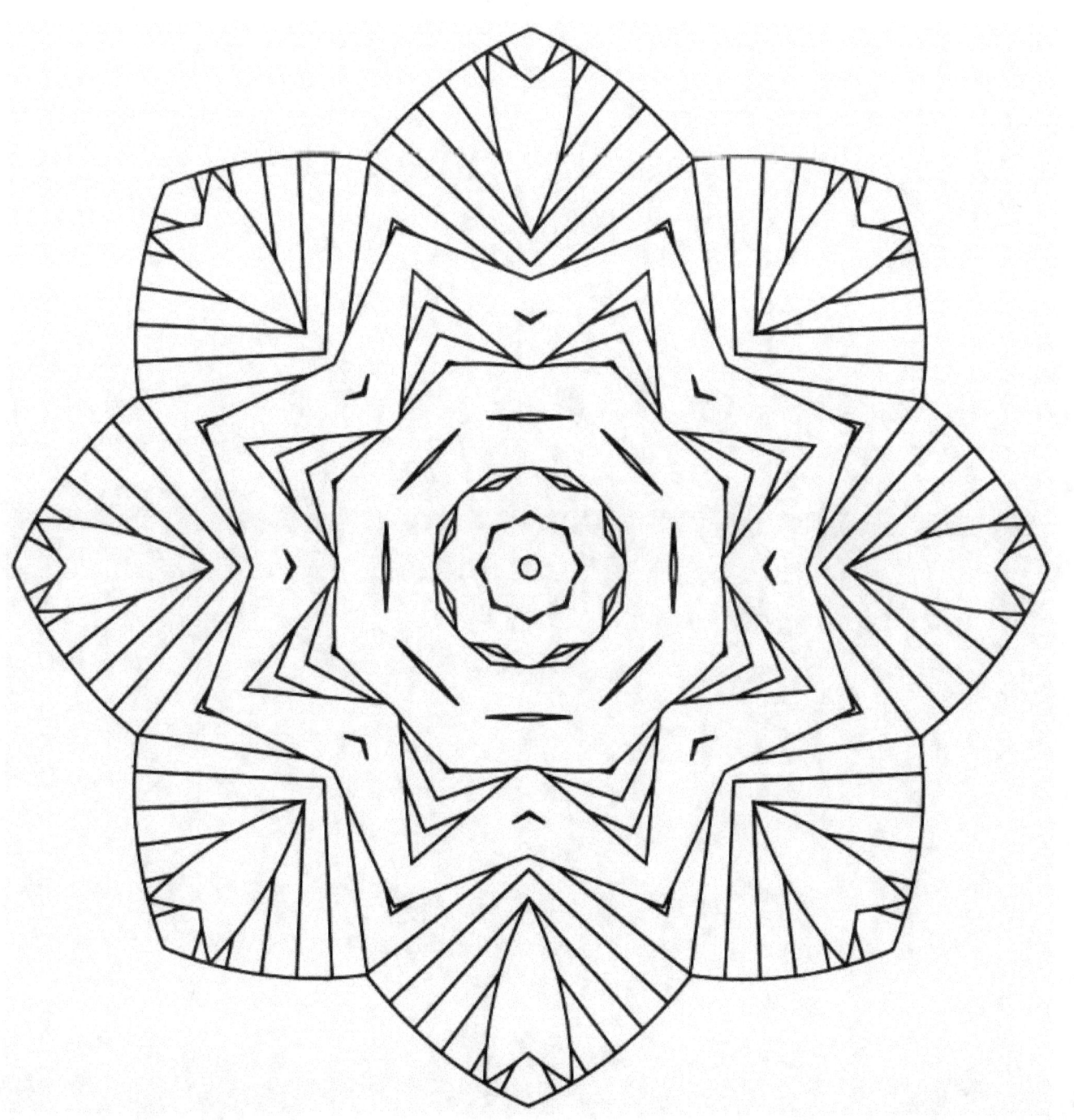

*There will never be a
perfect time to do
anything.
The time to take action is
now!*

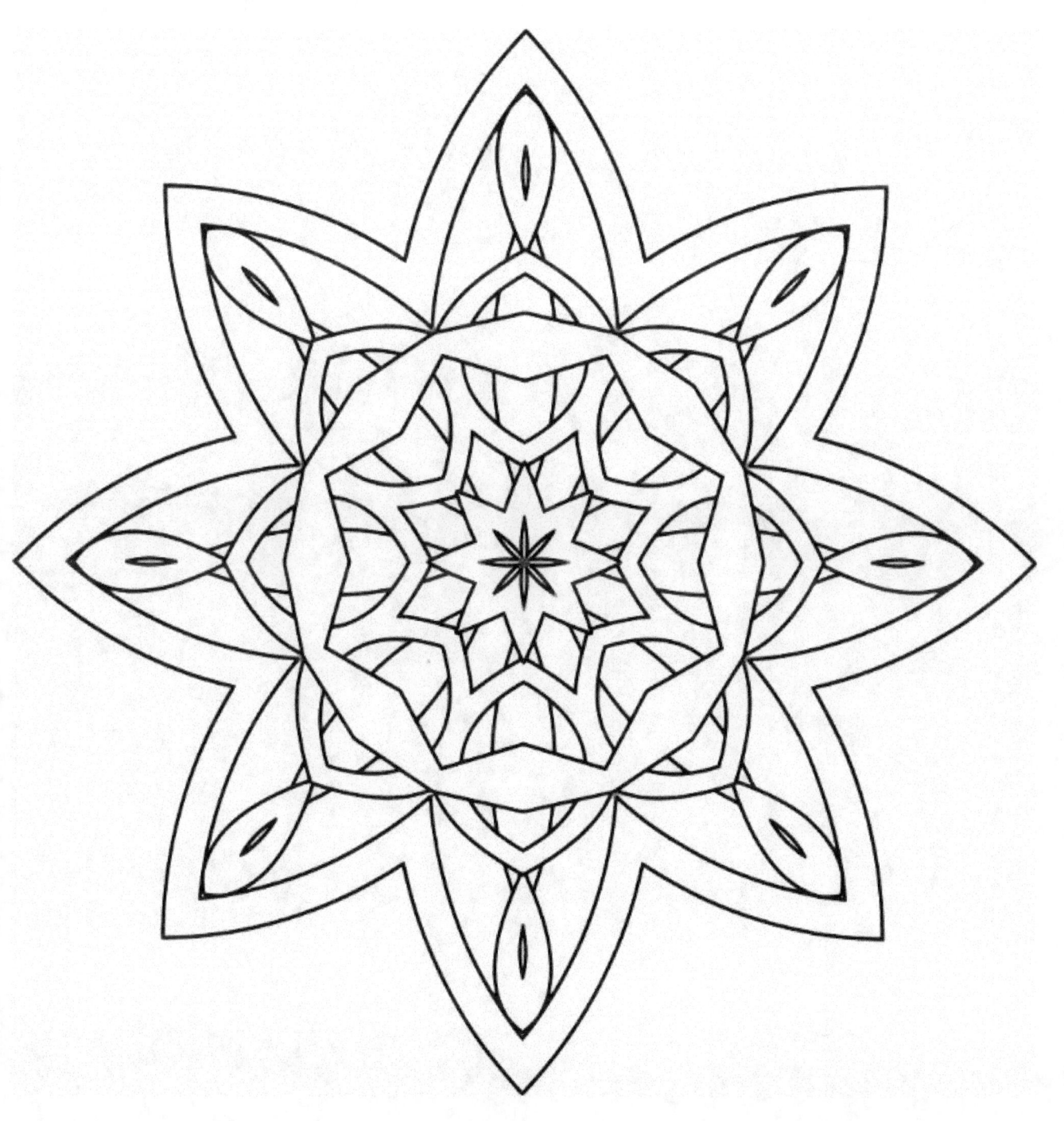

This feeling will pass;
I am ok!

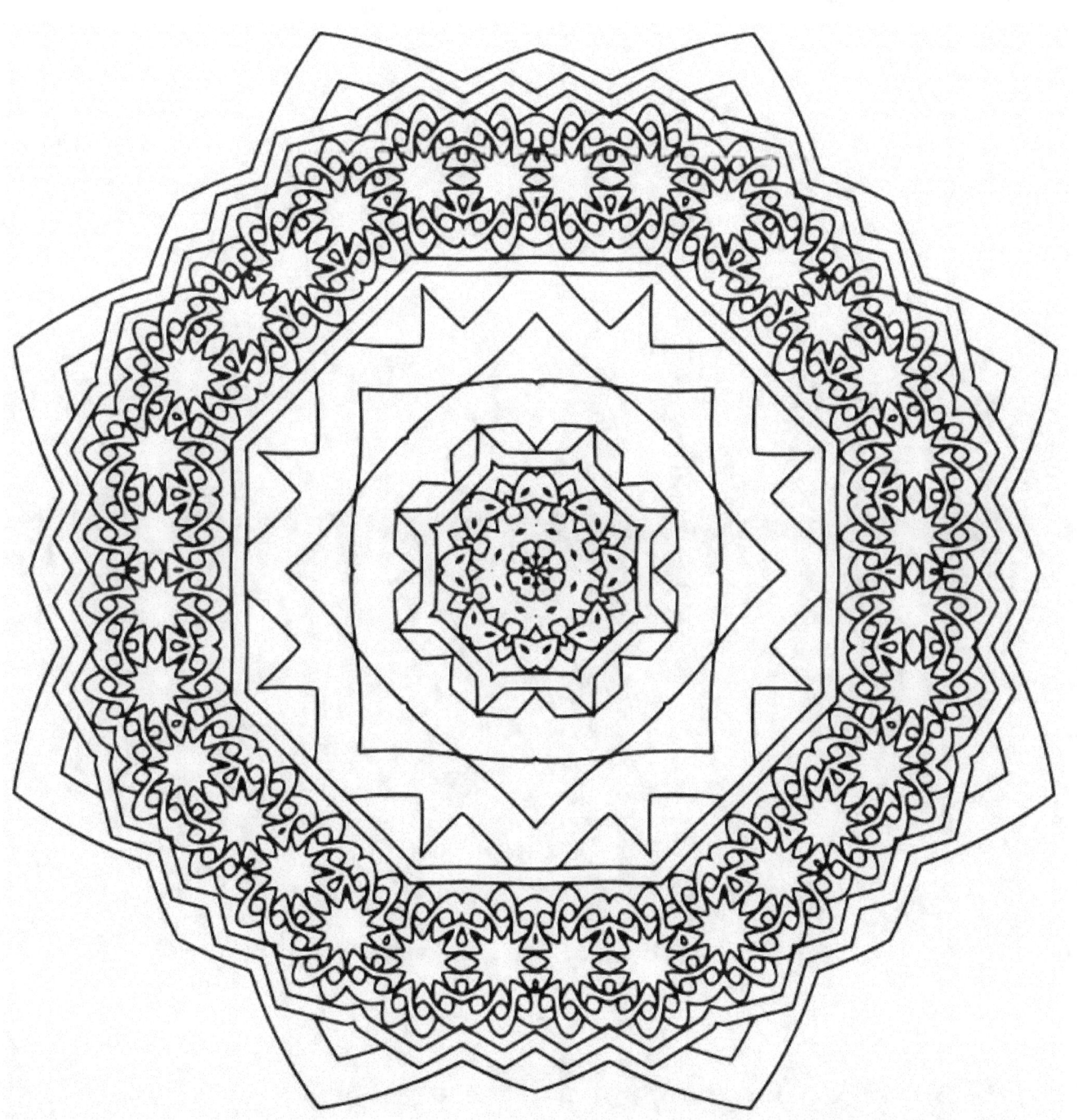

My life is a work in progress!

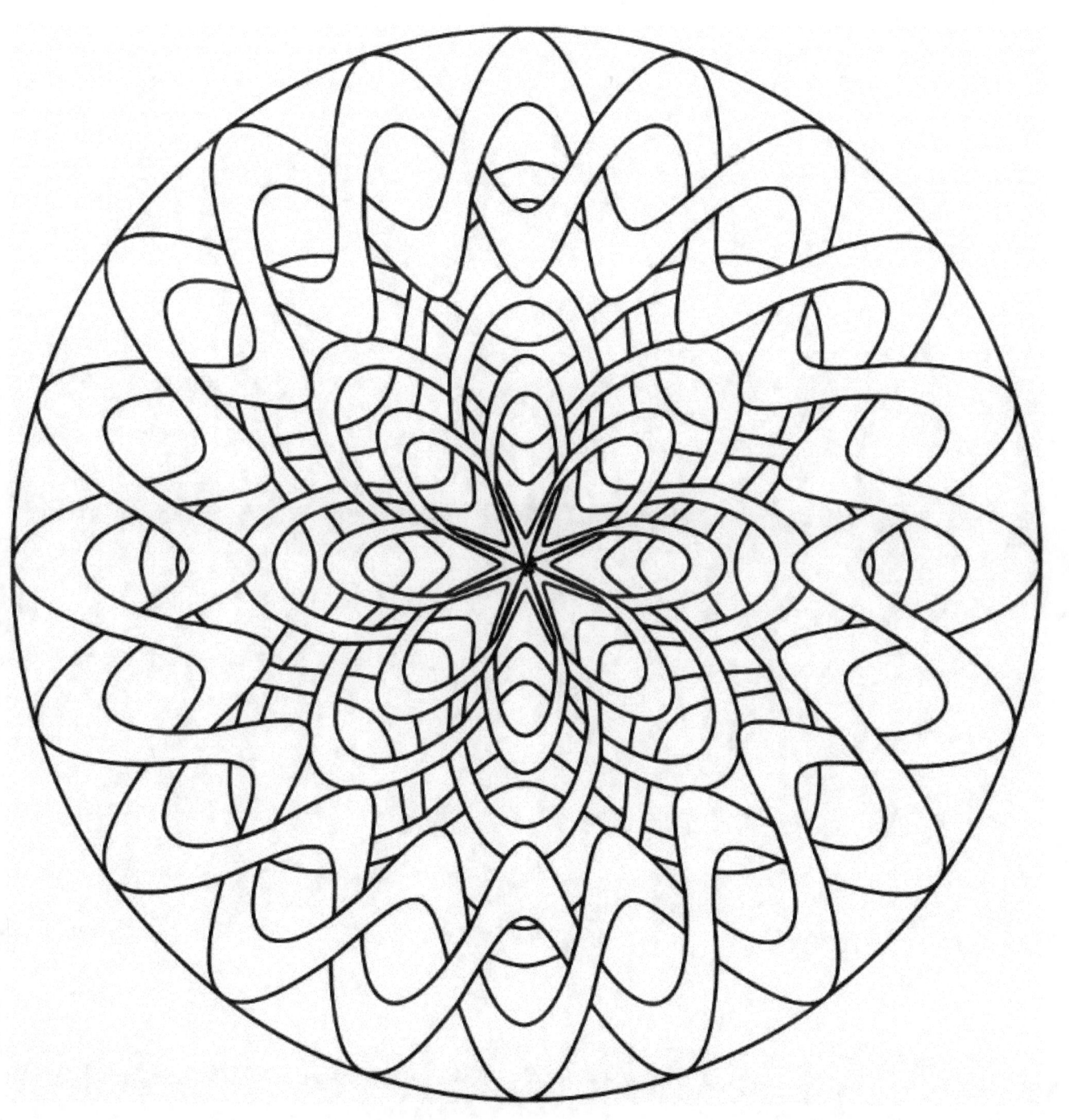

"There is little you can
learn from doing
nothing."

Zig Ziglar

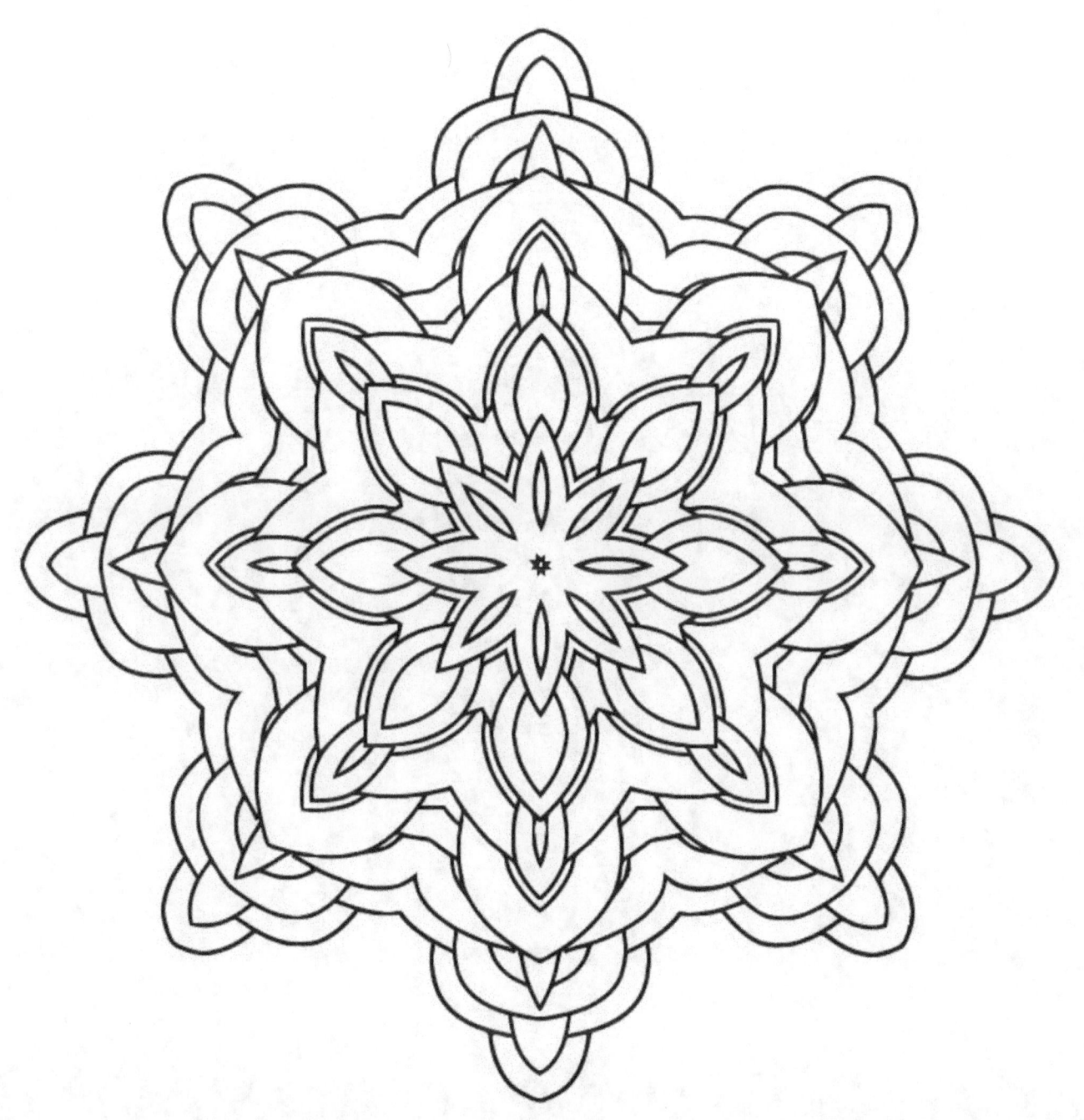

"Getting knocked down in life is a given. Getting up and moving forward is a choice."

Zig Ziglar

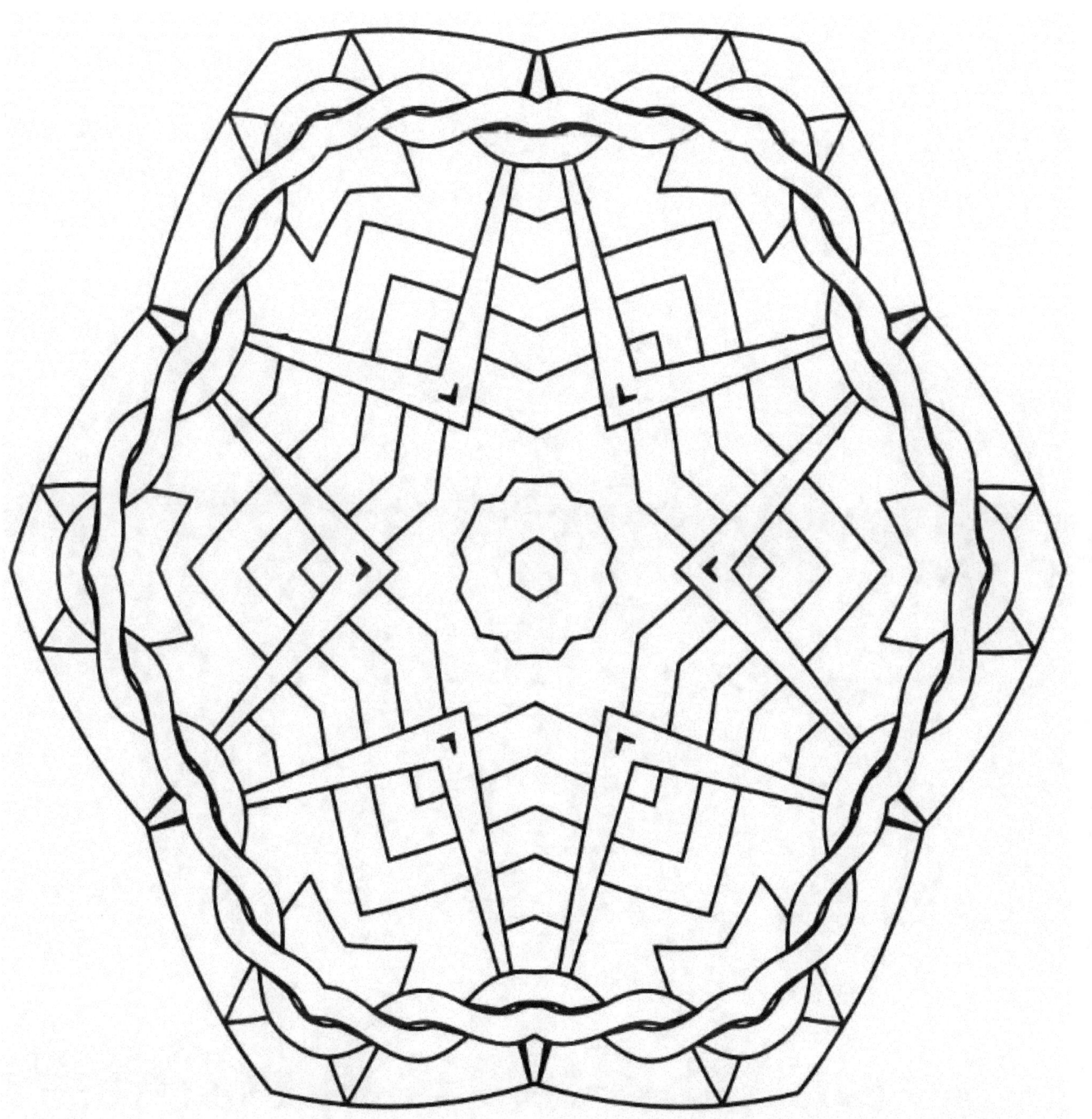

*To change your body,
you must first change
your mind!*

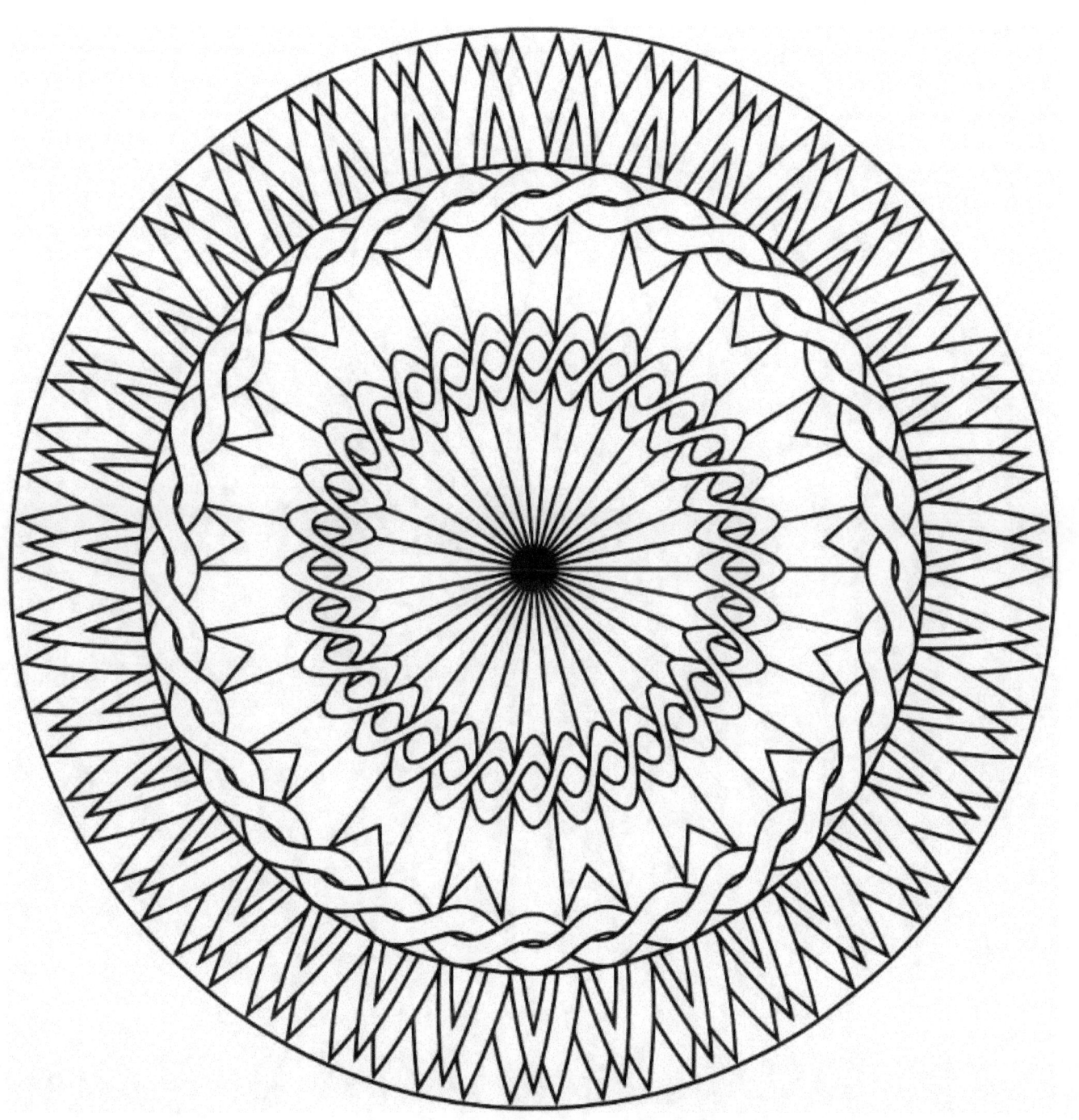

Sometimes it's ok if the
only thing you did today
is Breathe!

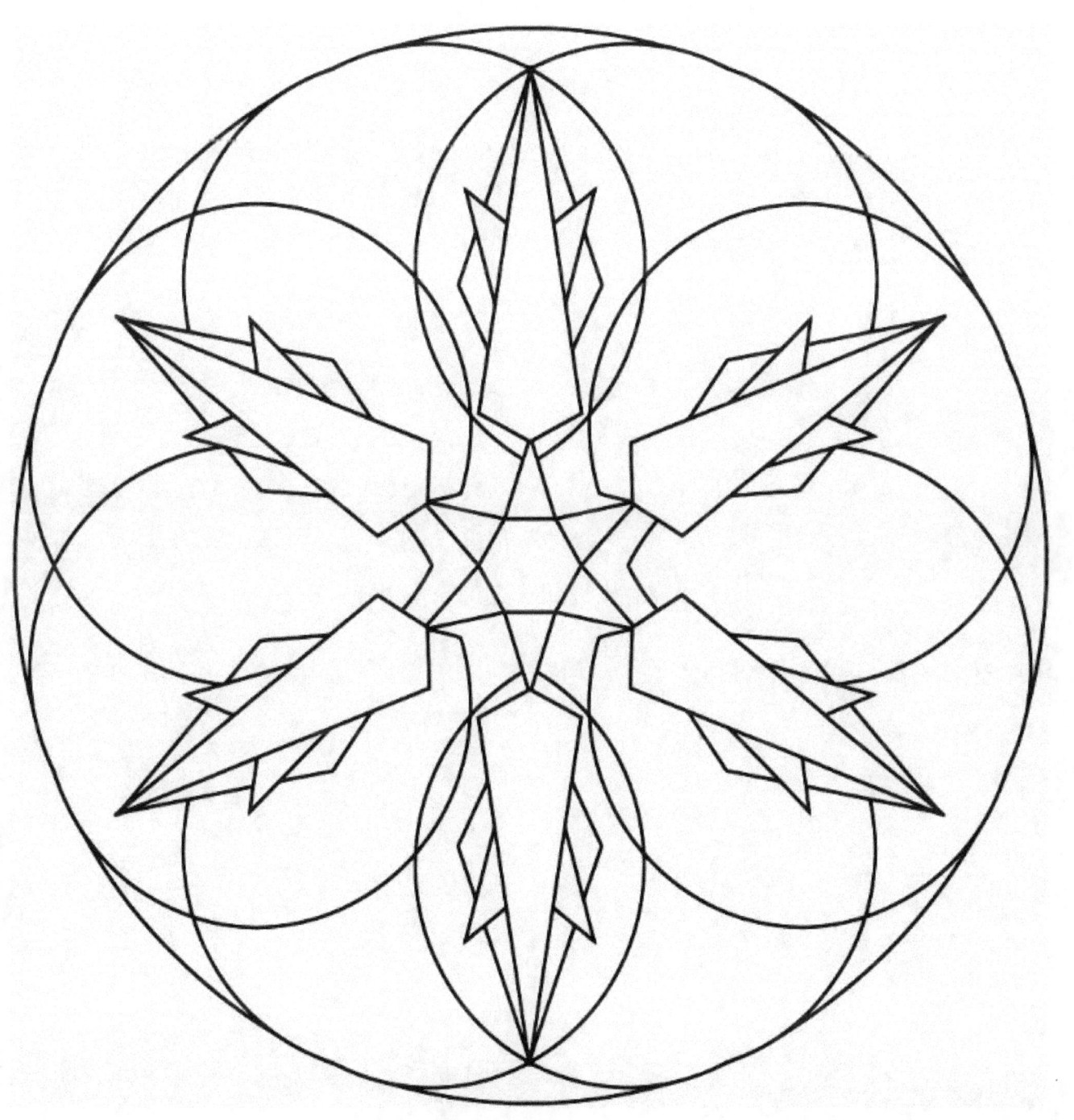

Don't just dream away
your life,
go out and start living
your dreams.

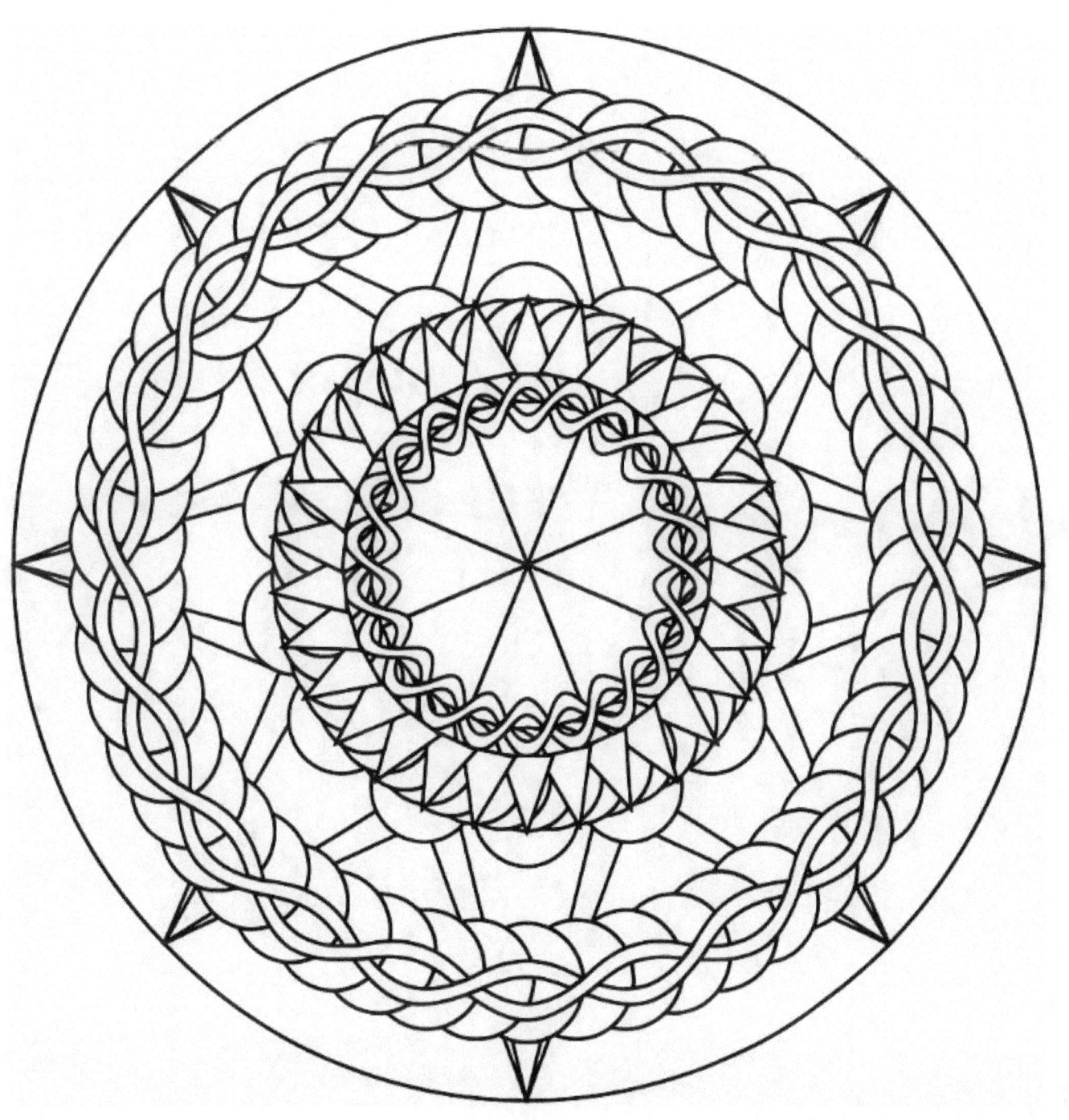

"Every choice you make
has an end result."

Zig Ziglar

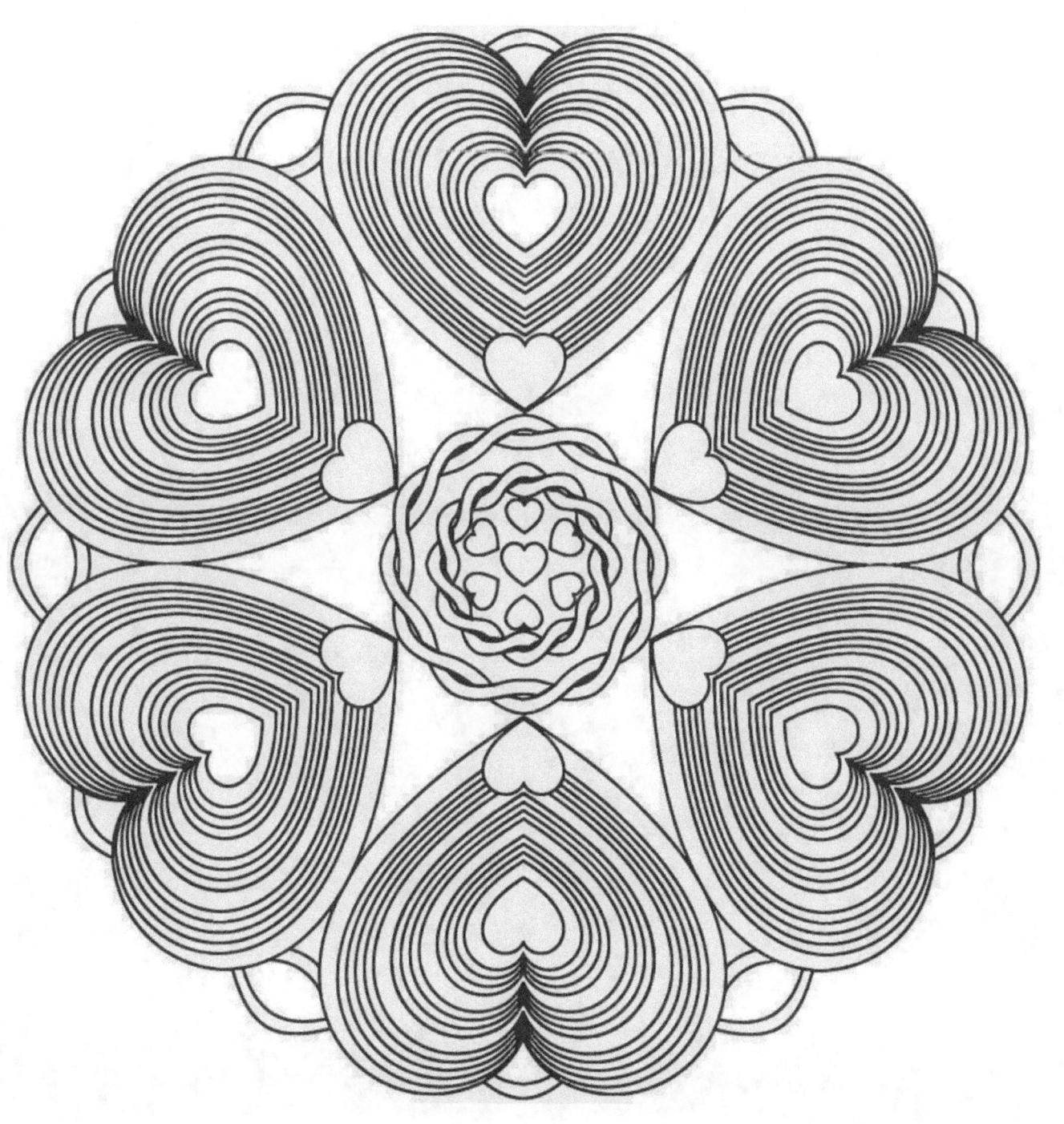

Don't waste energy
worrying about
things you can't control!

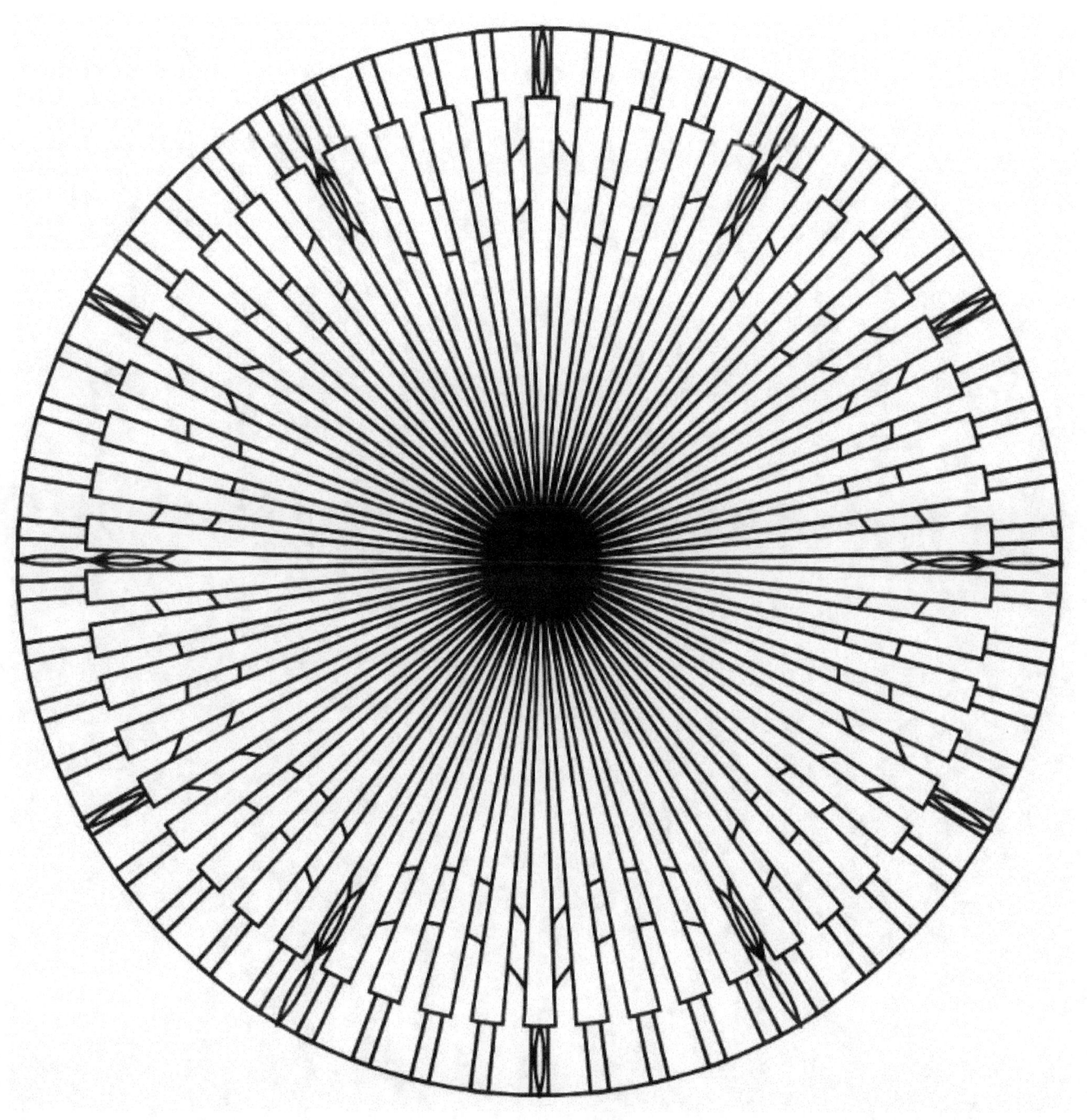

Every ending has a new beginning!

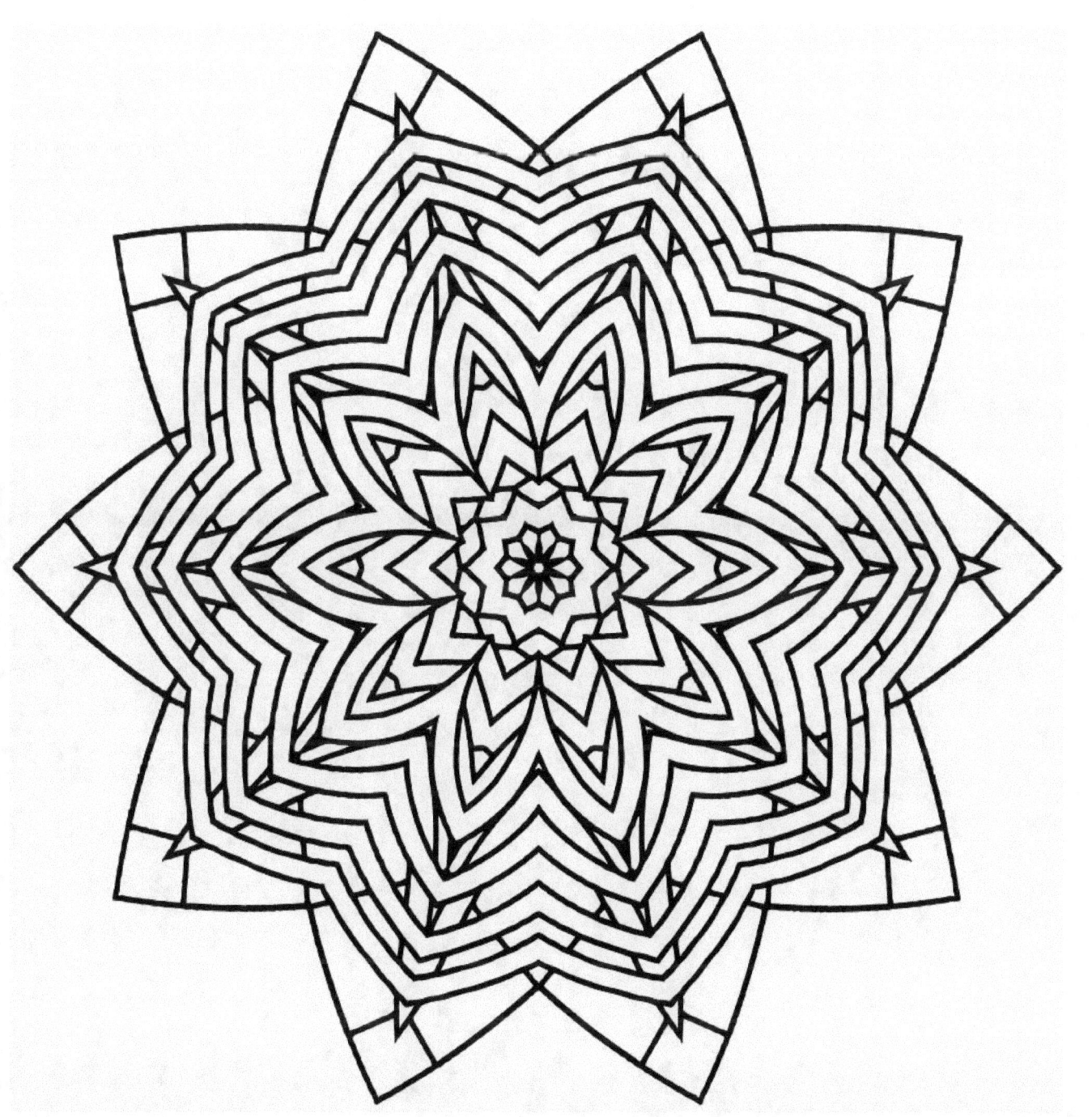

"Doing your best is more important than being the best."

Zig Ziglar

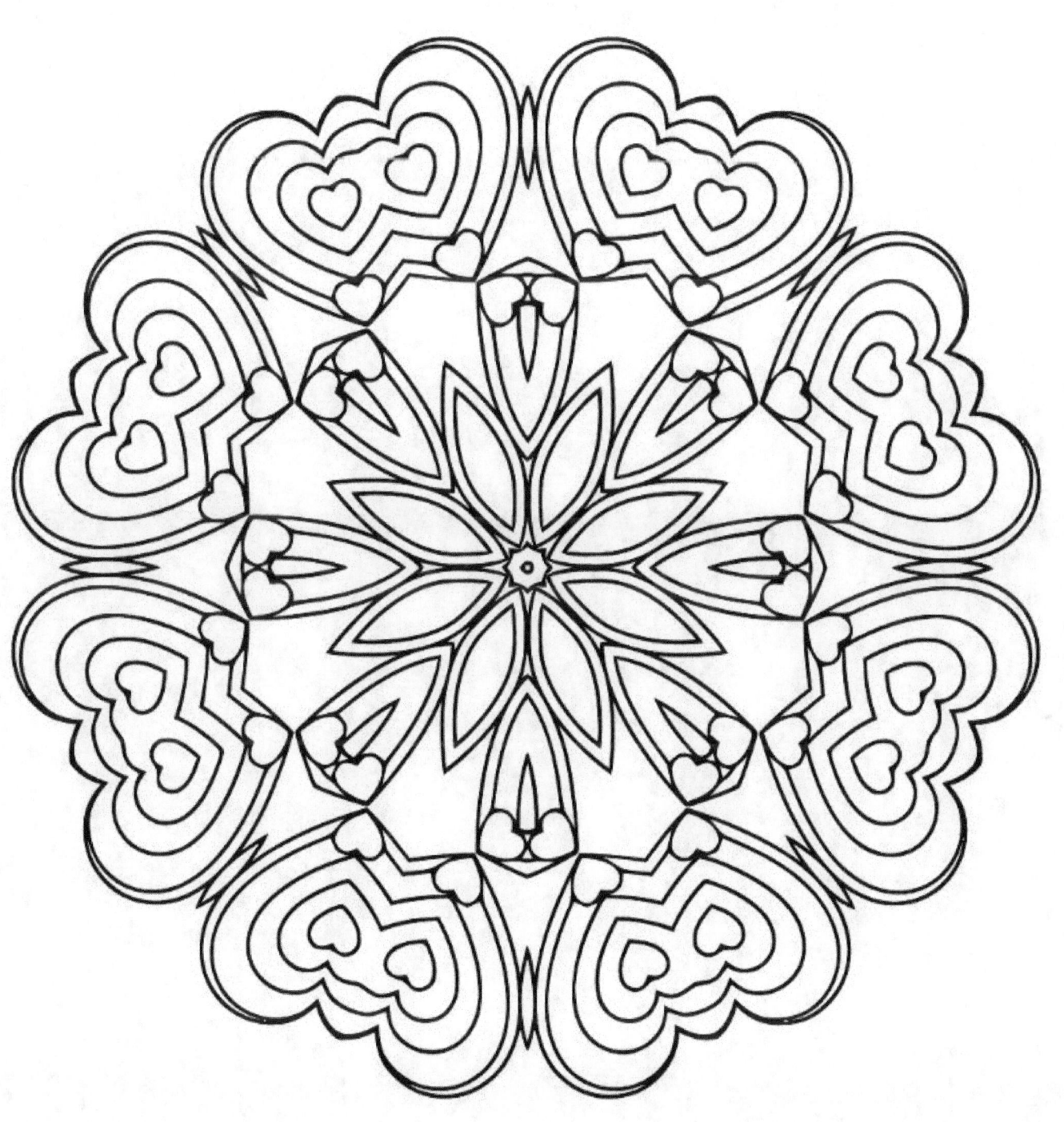

I love the person that I am!

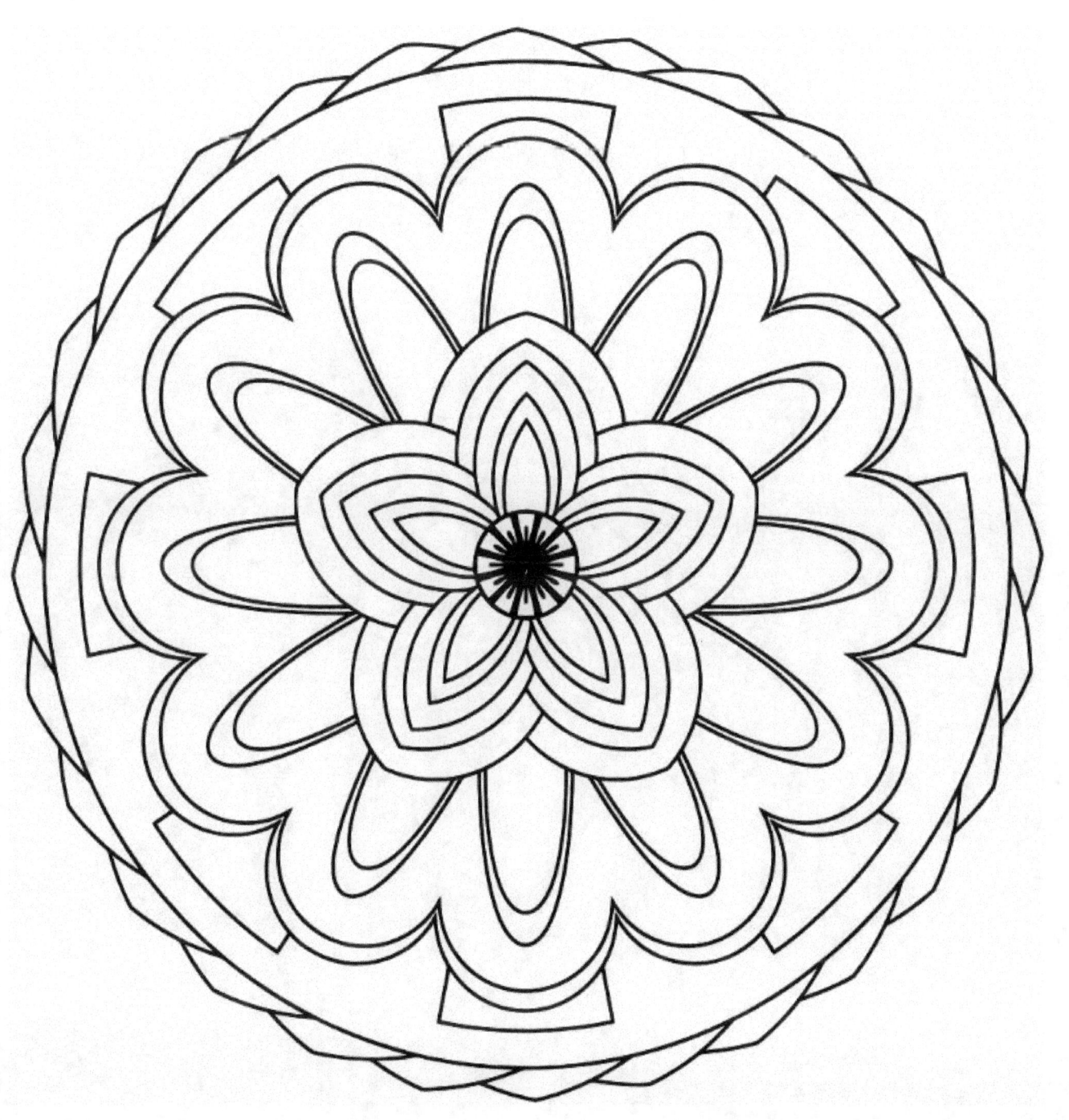

"Make today worth remembering."

Zig Ziglar

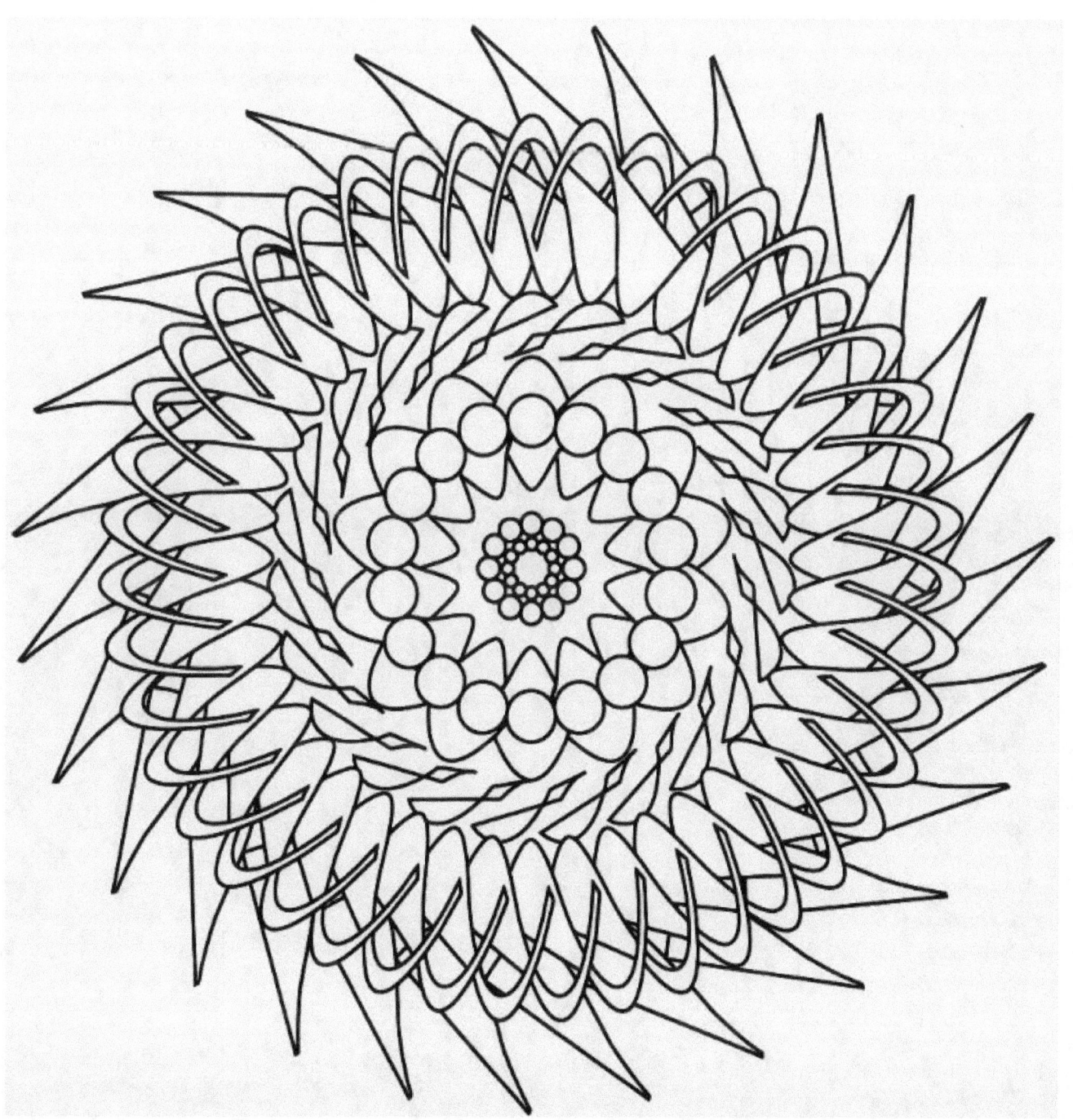

*Sometimes what you're
most afraid of doing,
is the very thing that will
set you free!*

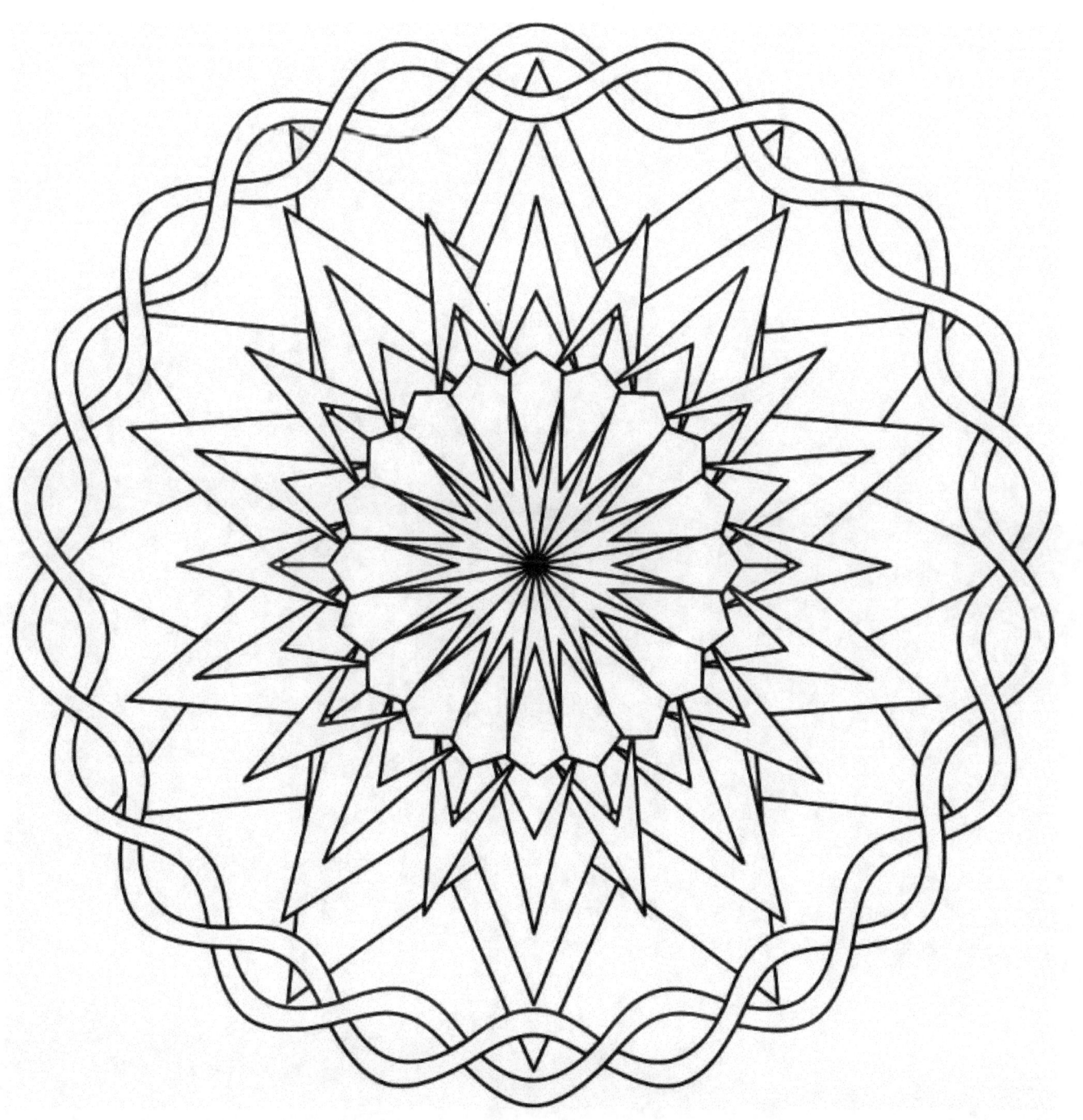

"Lack of direction, not lack of time is the problem.
We all have 24 hour days."

Zig Ziglar

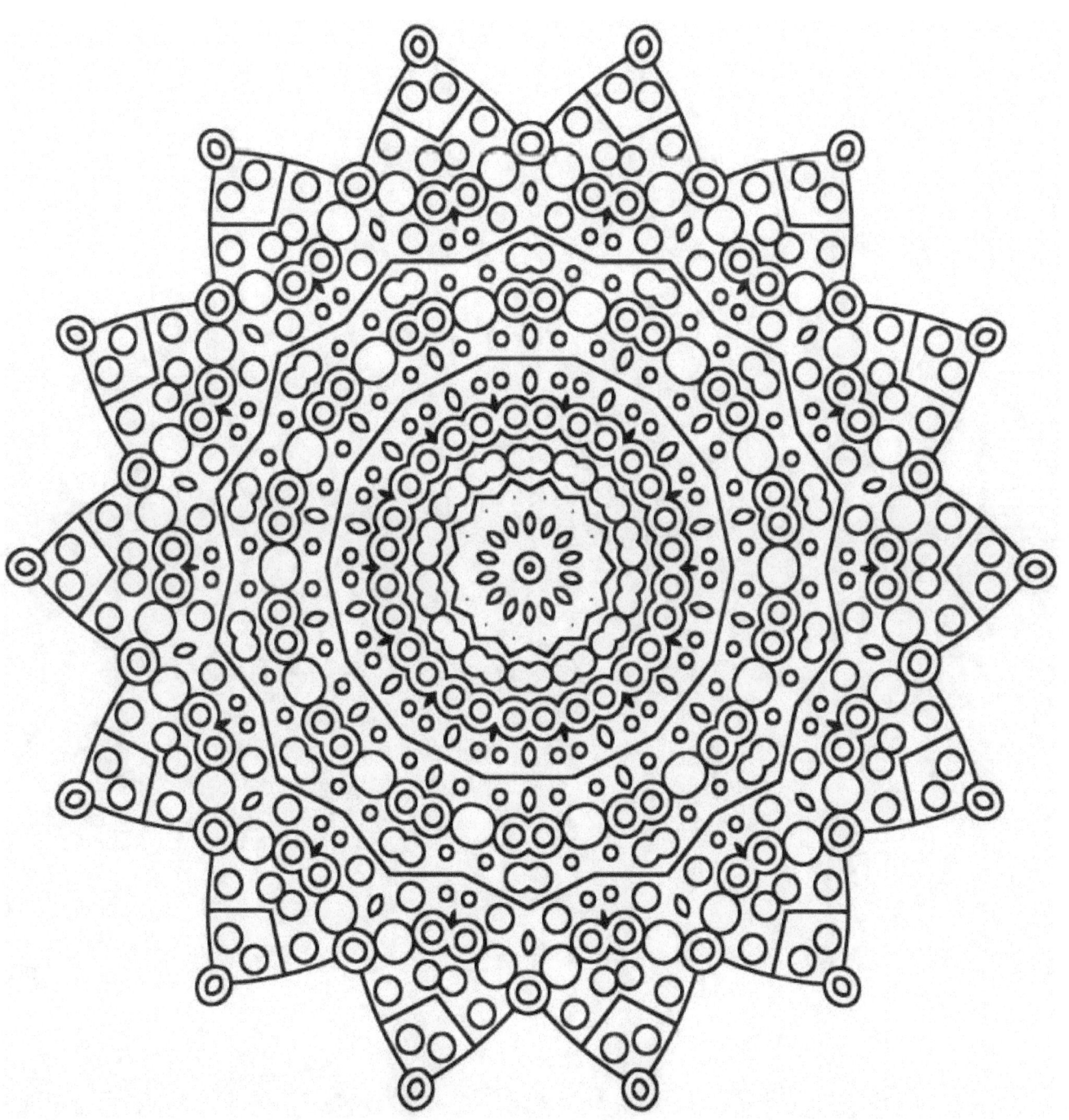

No matter how much you
revisit the past,
there is nothing new to
see!

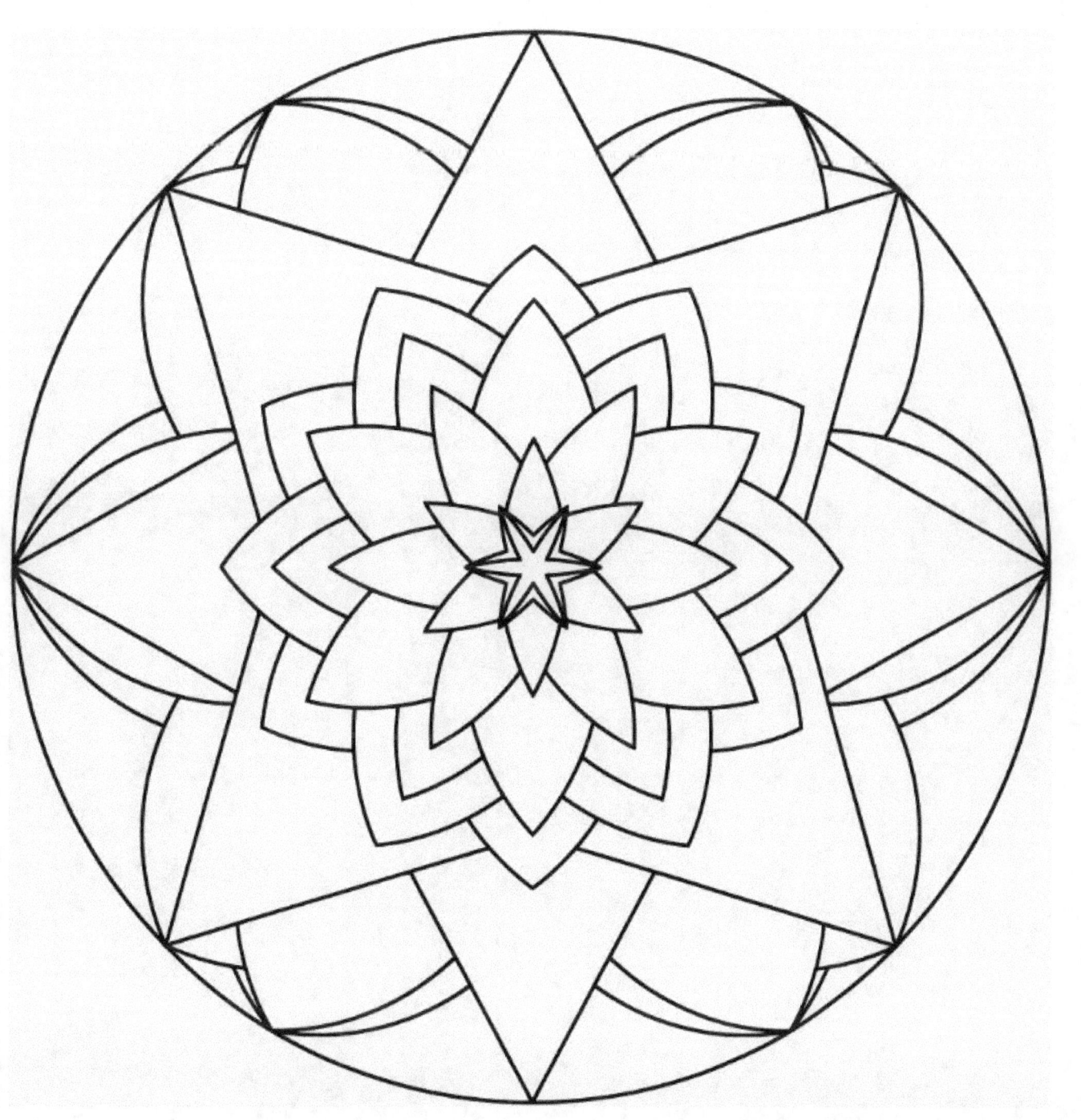

*"Remember that failure is
an event, not a person."*

Zig Ziglar

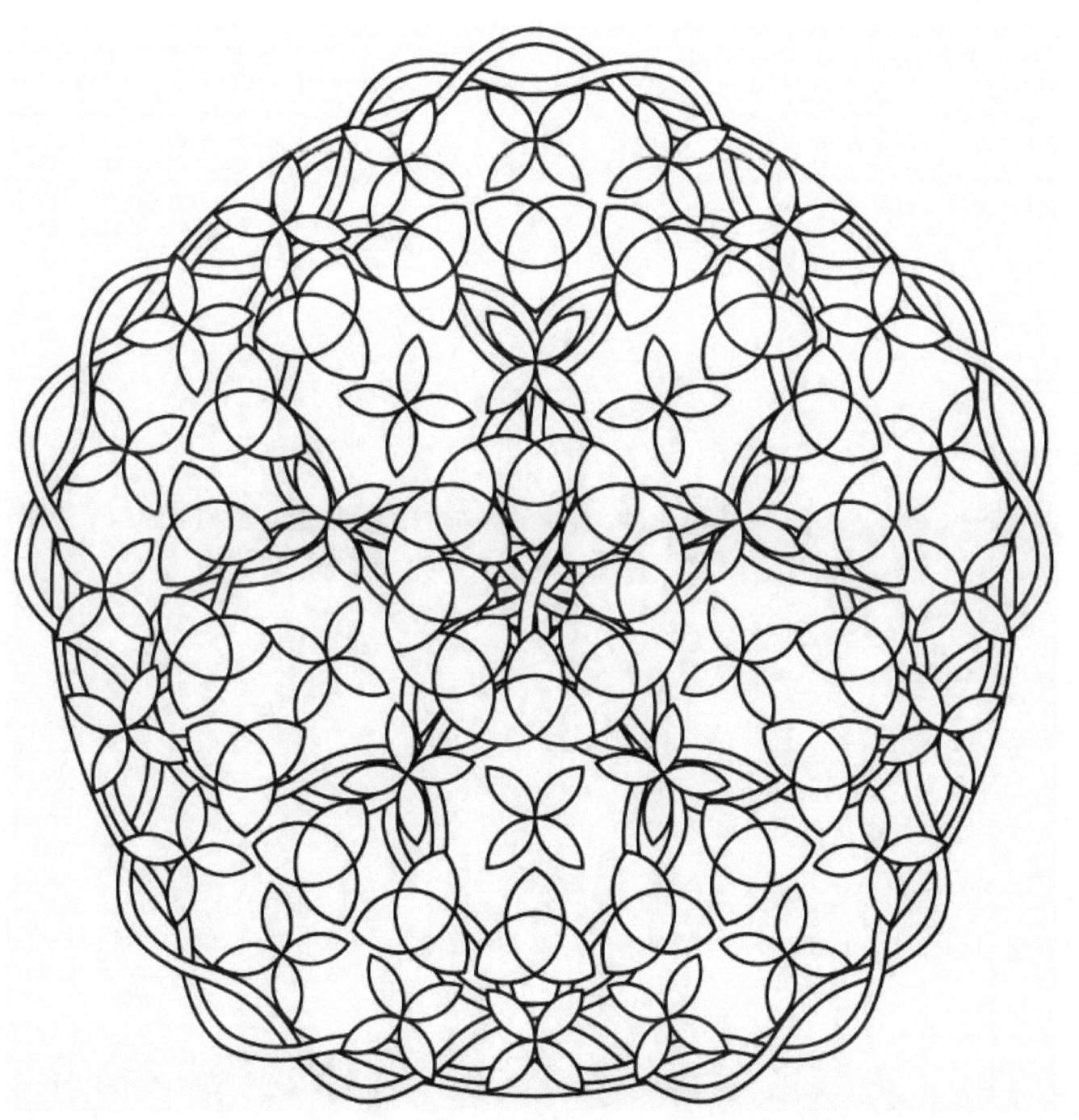

A flower doesn't compete
with the one next to it
– it just blooms.

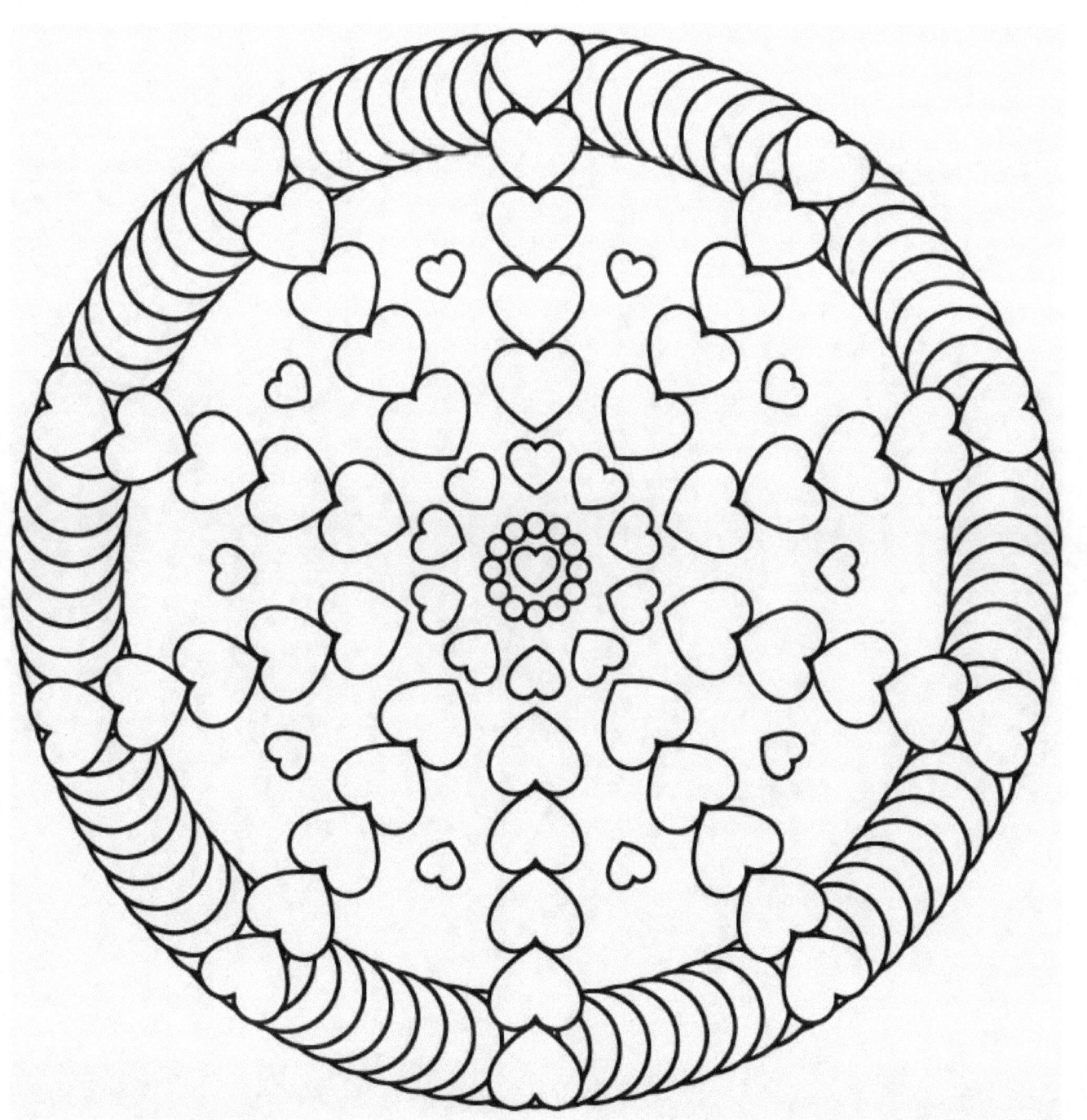

Laughter is the best medicine!

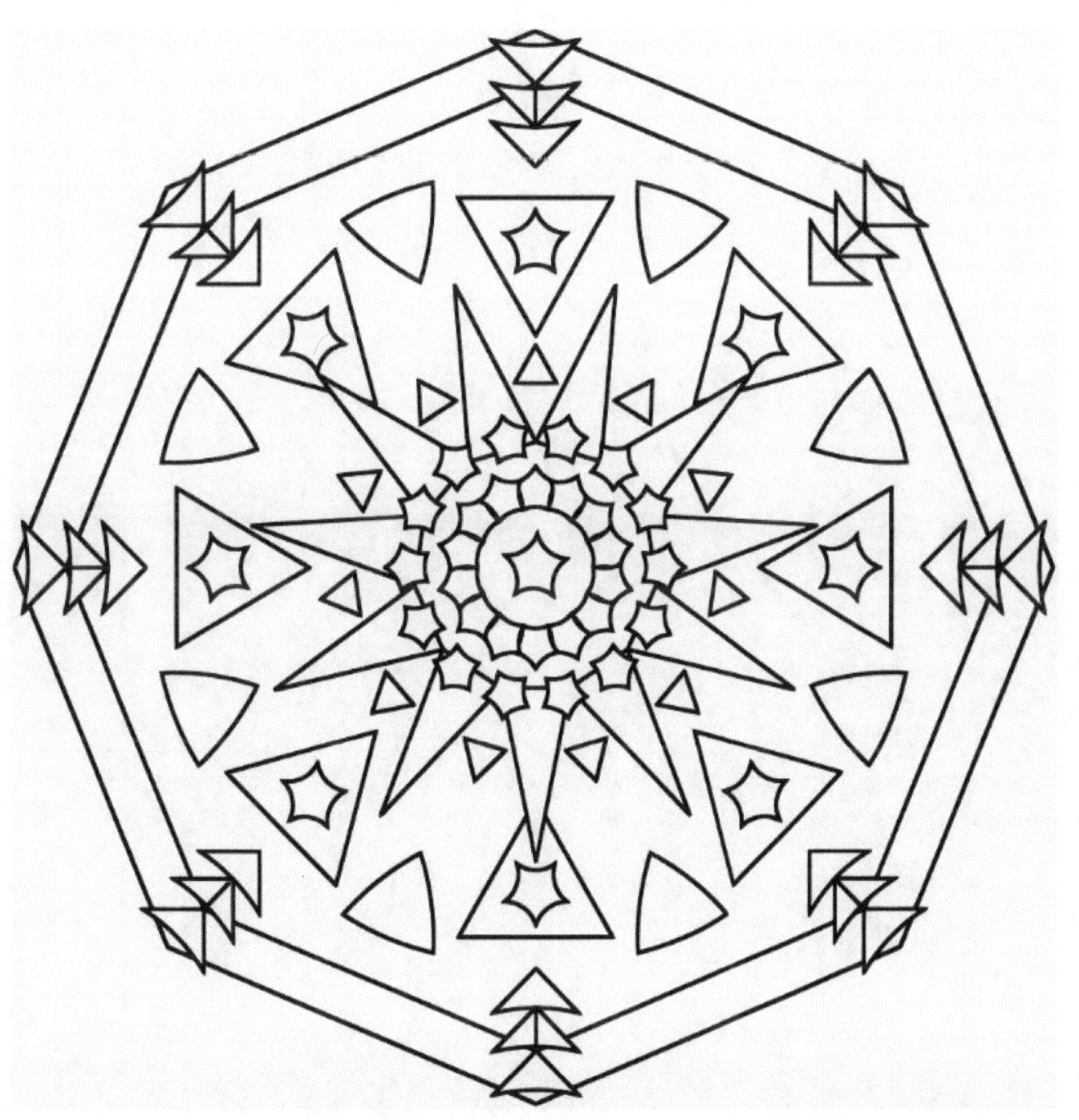

Don't dwell on the past,
just keep moving forward!

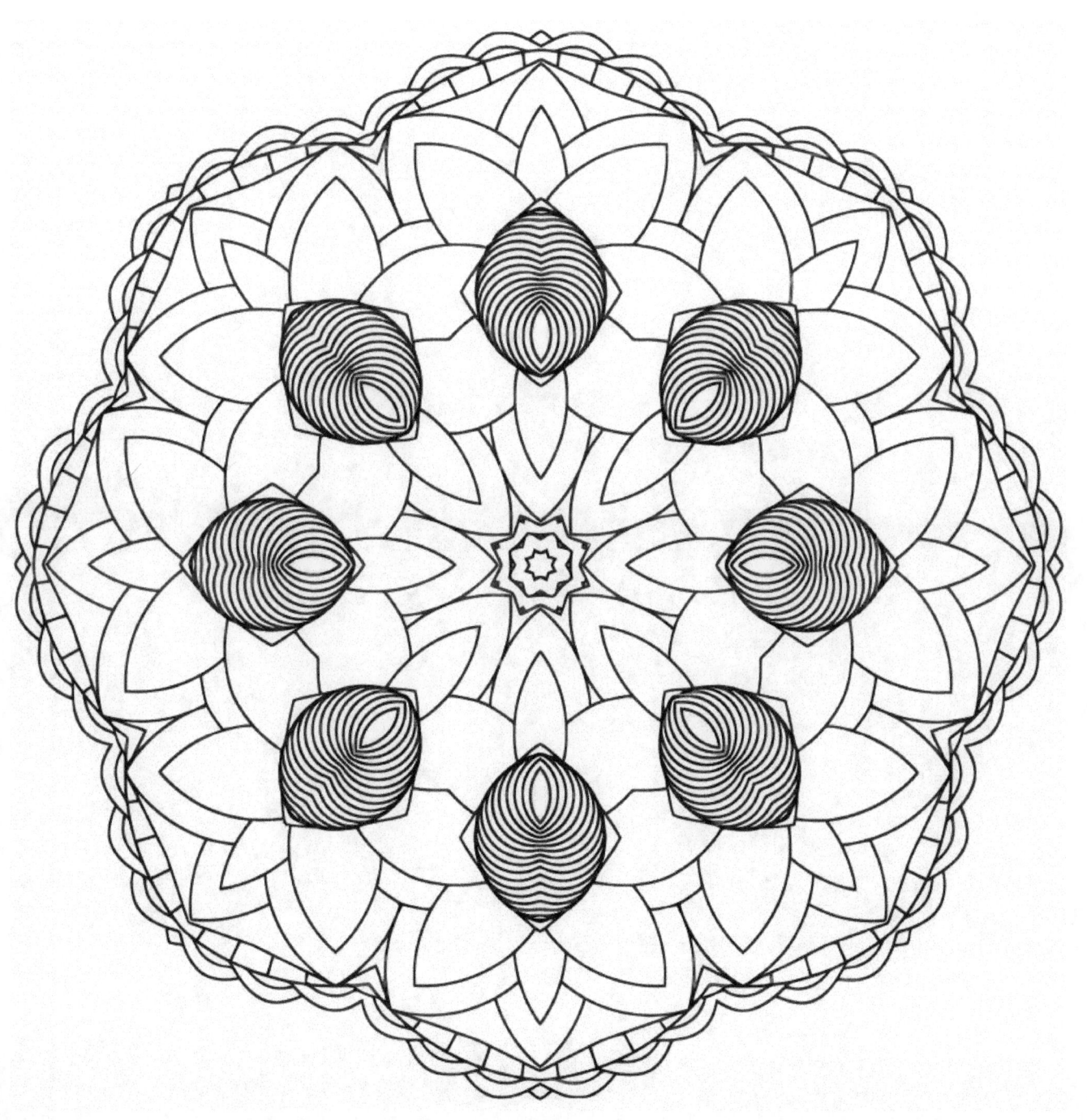

Remind yourself that it's
ok not to be perfect.

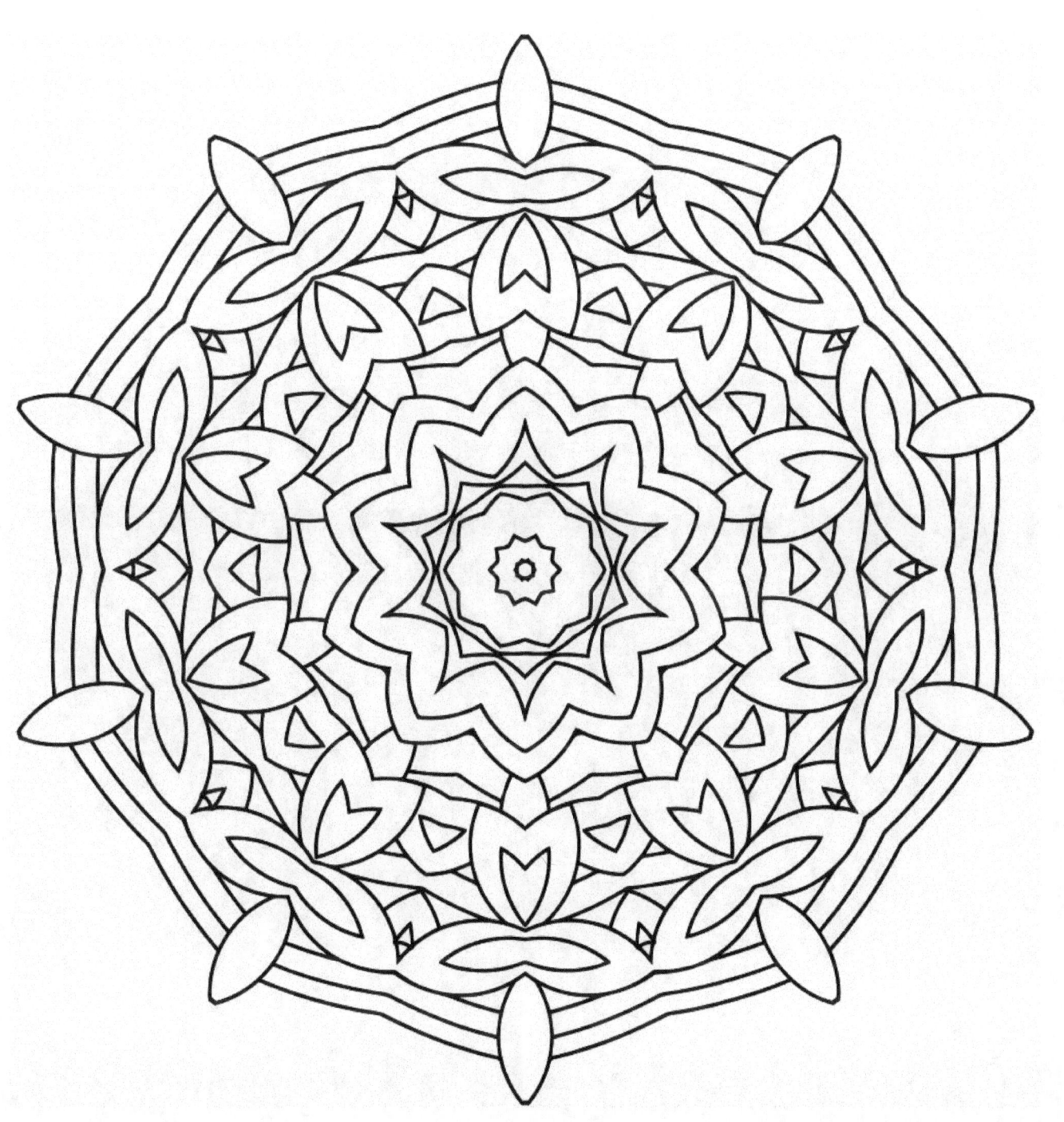

Practice thinking positive
because it can change
your life!

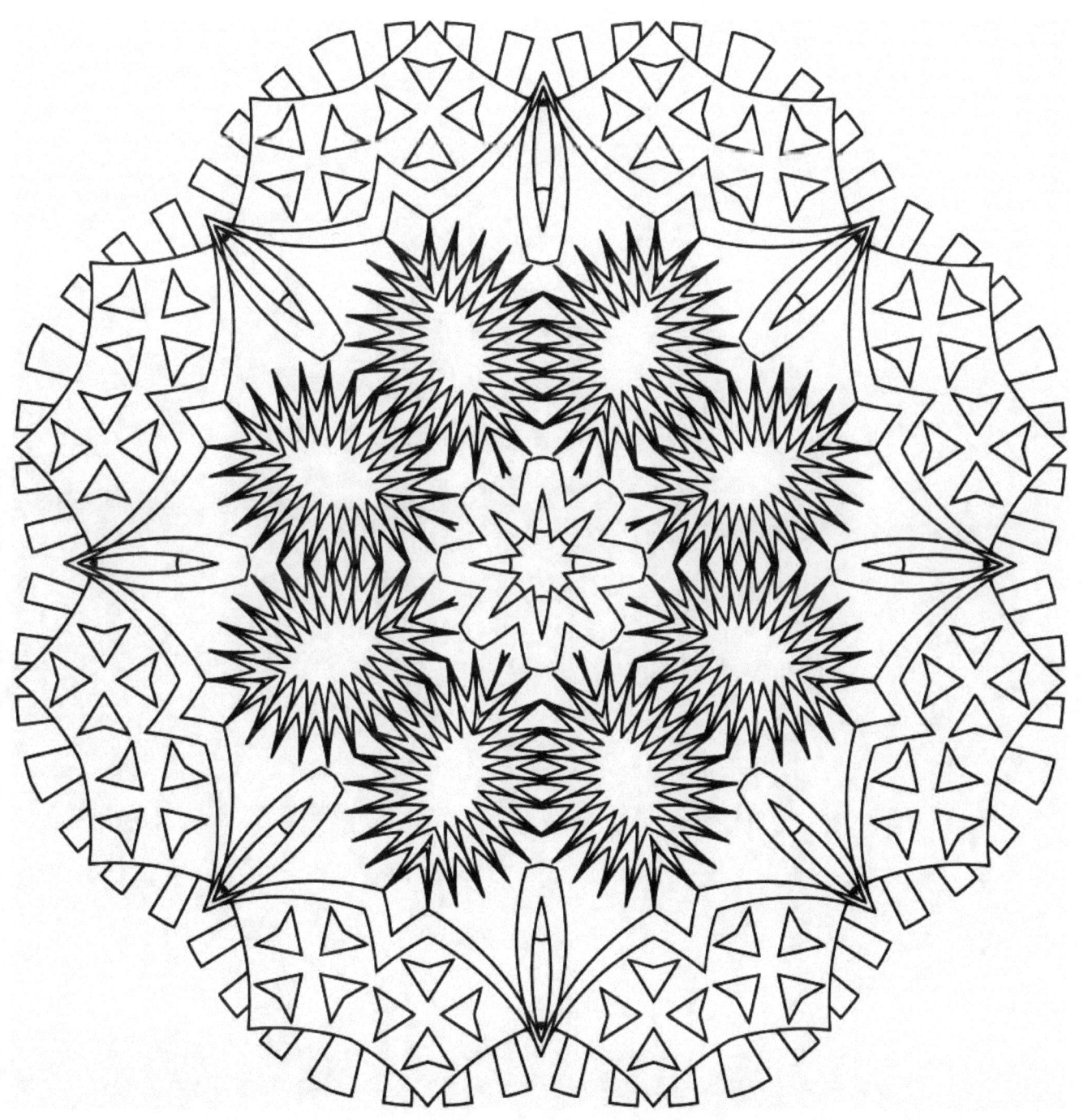

*One of the happiest
moments in life,
is when you find the
courage
to let go of what you
cannot change.*

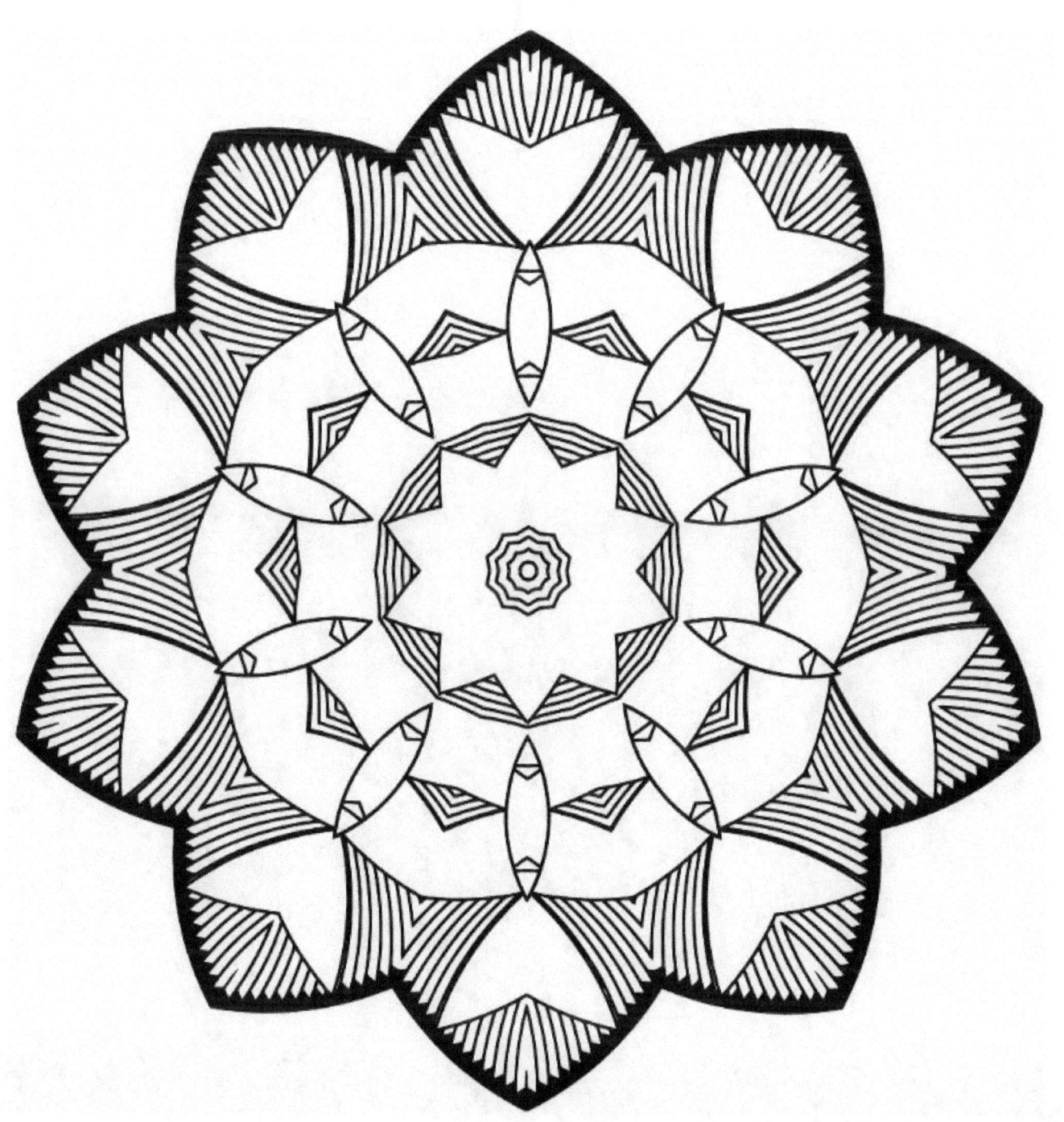

*Life is a balance of holding
on and letting go!*

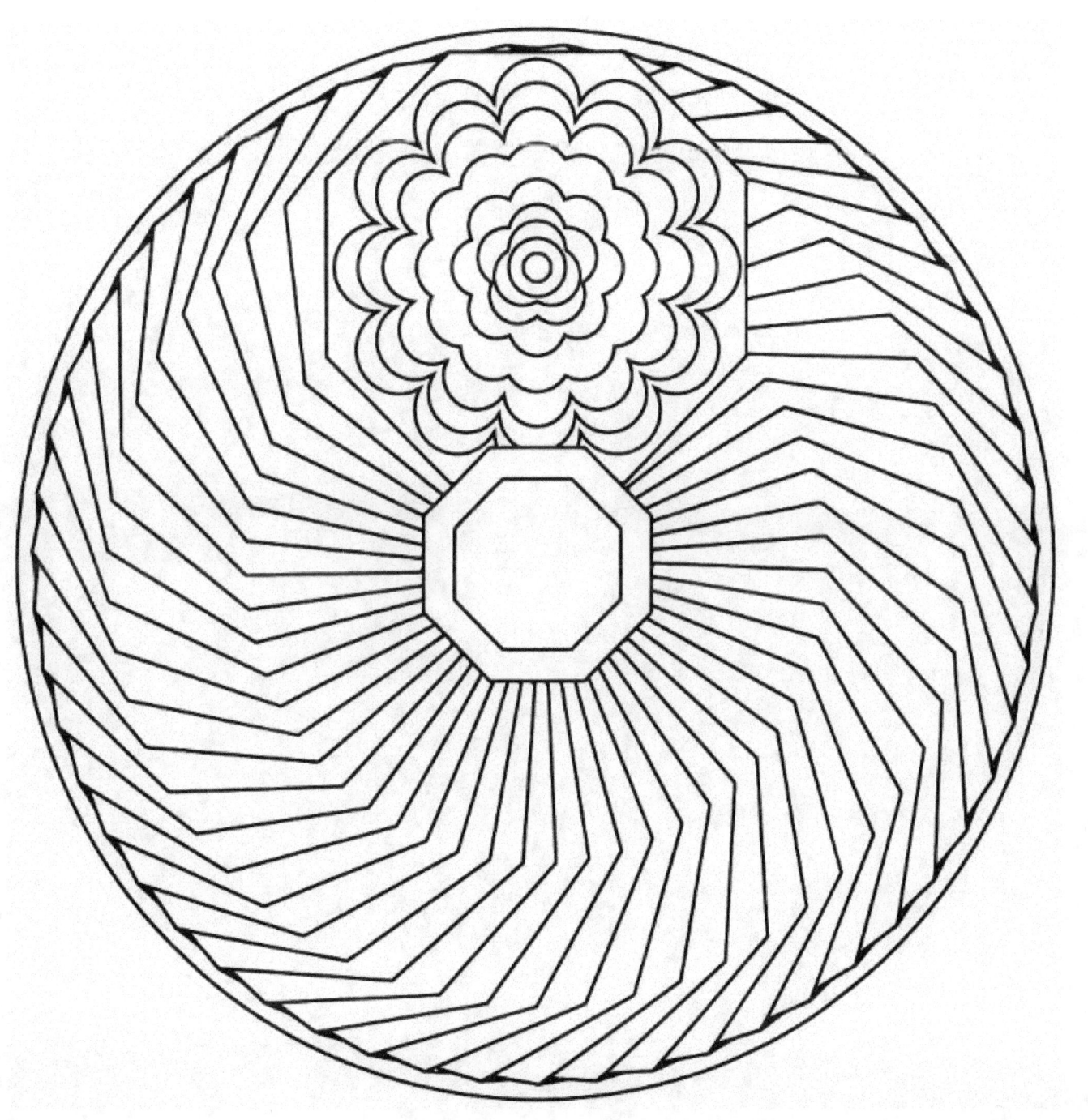

Surround yourself with positive people!

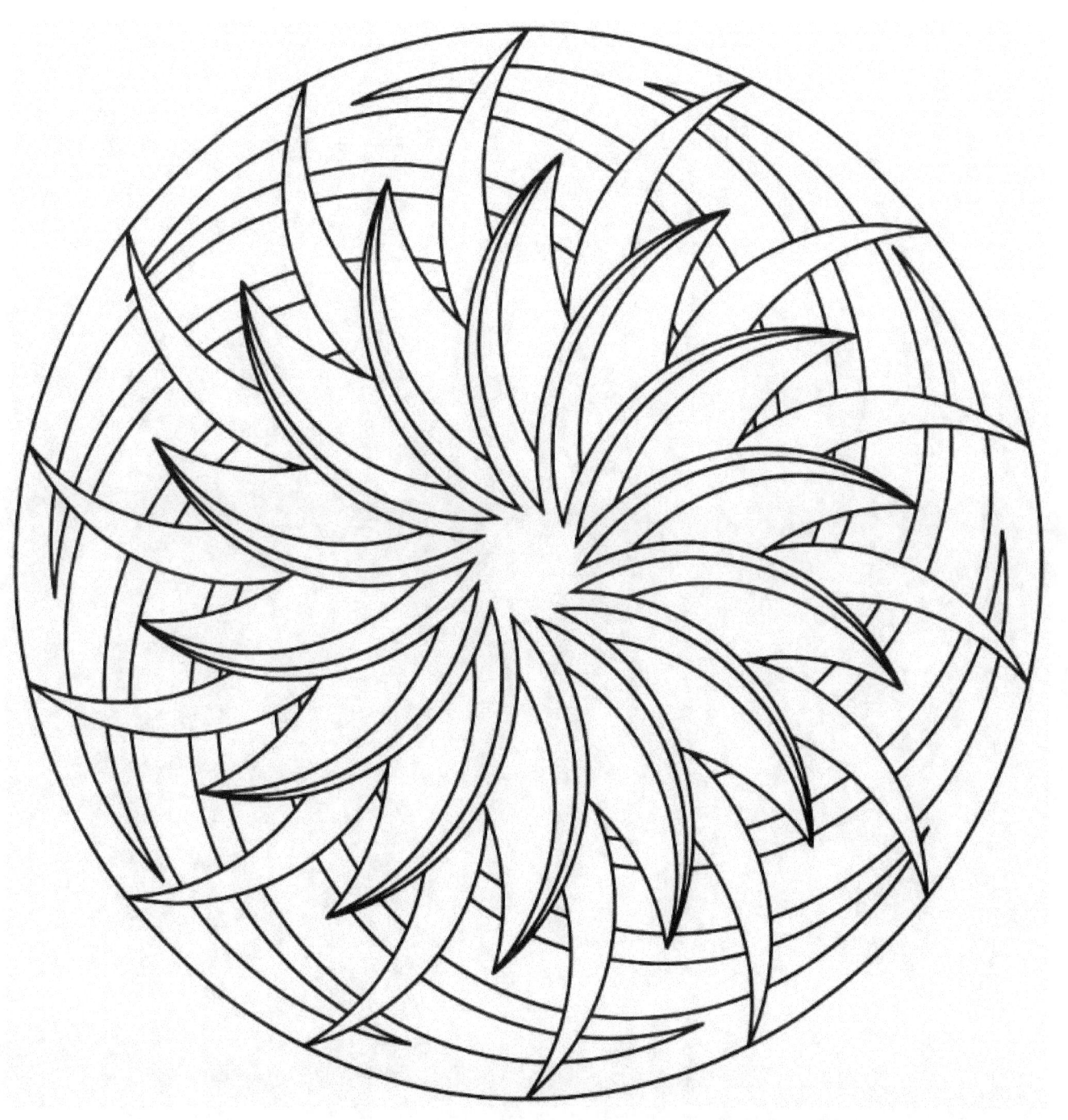

Stay In Touch & Explore More!

I hope you have enjoyed coloring this book and ask if you would please take just a moment to leave an honest review of my coloring book either on Etsy or Amazon.

I would also like to invite you to check out all of my Adult Coloring Books that are available as a paperback from Amazon here: https://amzn.to/2OK28P6 or as a PDF Digital download from my Etsy store here: https://www.etsy.com/au/shop/ColorYourWayToHappy

I love being creative and with over 40 books published so far, I'm always adding new books each month so be sure to check back and see if there's something you like.

Alternatively, if you would like to be kept up-to-date with new book releases and news please take the time to visit my Facebook page and feel free to let your friends and family know about my page too.

Don't forget to like and comment on my page and you're welcome to share your colored pages from my books there too!

Just go to: www.facebook.com/ColorYourWayToHappy

Thanks again and remember to have fun and go 'Color Your Way To Happy'!

Nerine ☺

www.ingramcontent.com/pod-product-compliance
Lightning Source LLC
Chambersburg PA
CBHW080601180526
45168CB00007B/2740